LOVE, DIGNITY
&
PARKINSON'S

from Care Partner to Caregiver

by Terri Pease, Ph.D.

Publishing Services provided by Paper Raven Books LLC

Published by Seabury House Press LLC

Printed in the United States of America

First Printing, 2022

Paperback ISBN: 979-8-9867001-0-6

Large Print ISBN: 979-8-9867001-1-3

DISCLAIMER:
The information, including but not limited to, text, graphics, images and other material contained in this book are for informational purposes only. No material is intended to be a substitute for professional medical advice, diagnosis, or treatment. Always seek the advice of your physician or another qualified healthcare provider with any questions you may have regarding a medical condition or treatment before under-taking a new healthcare regimen.

To my husband, Peter.

"…together even in the silent memory of God."
Khalil Gibran

Special Offers

A s a bonus for readers of *Love, Dignity and Parkinson's*, I have designed a printable workbook and journal that contains the check-in questions for each chapter, with space to write your thoughts and ideas as you go along.

Scan the QR code below to get your access to this and other resources.

Contents

Acknowledgements

Looking back on all the supportive people who were in my life during my years of caregiving leaves my heart full.

Of course, there was my family, and especially my girls. My own Rebecca— my lifeline—who I could always count on for a phone call or text chat at any time, no matter how busy her family and work life had made her.

Peter's daughters, the other Rebecca and Francesca, who became my daughters too, were fellow travelers along this path. They had been caring for their father before he and I ever met, gracefully acknowledged our loving partnership, and made room for me to become his wife and primary caregiver.

Kelley Roberson and the Parkinson's Better Halves community (pbh-org.com) and Jim Smitchger, founder of myParkinsons.org, gave me a community of other caregivers to sustain me when things were hard and encouraged my contributions to their communities as well. I found my first readers of an early draft of this book there—thank you all for the helpful suggestions, which improved this book so much.

We were so lucky to know the founders, staff, families, and housemates of The Mooring on Foreside. Lynn Peel, how did you happen to open your wonderful community just when we needed you?

Dr. Erin Shaw-Nkurunziza, OT extraordinaire, was an important early advocate for self-care, while helping Peter in so many ways. The other medical providers, therapists, and home helpers who cared so well for my husband and for me are too many to list, for fear that I'll leave out someone important. Thank you all. You know how you've helped.

Althea Rosenbloom, thank you—you, too, know how you've helped—always.

Most especially, I thank the many Parkinson's Caregivers—in person and in online groups and forums—whose shared experience and wisdom help all of us caregivers sustain ourselves and our love for our PWPs.

My work on this book has benefitted from so very many people that I am sure to leave someone out. So please forgive me if I'm not expressing my thanks here, and know, as you already do, that you helped as well, and that I am indeed grateful.

Thanks to Joshua Sprague, who got me started on writing this book and made me believe that it could be done, and to John DeDakis, who helped me learn how to do it.

As Peter used to say, "This thing was too important to be rushed."

Terri Pease

Yarmouth, Maine

Introduction

I'm going to guess that this is not the first book on Parkinson's Disease (PD) that you've picked up. Many partners of people with PD seek information as energetically as a student who's cramming for the SATs. And many times, PD partners are motivated by the instinctive sense that PD is not a one-person disease.

Long before the official diagnosis of PD, partners often notice that something is "off." PD's effects are not just physical. A loving partner often notices changes that can be both subtle and global. Many times, dopamine loss (the underlying cause of PD symptoms) affects a person's appearance and behavior long before the muscular and movement changes become evident enough to warrant a trip to a physician.

One thing that motivated me to write this book for Parkinson's partners was when I realized that as Parkinson's begins to rob a person's facial expressions and emotional responsiveness, their partner may assume that these changes signal a breakdown in their relationship. It's not unheard of for a wife to end her marriage in reaction to these changes in her husband, only to learn some years after splitting up that what looked like disconnection was dopamine loss instead.

So, if you have noticed that your PWP, your Partner with Parkinson's, no longer smiles as broadly, or doesn't respond as lovingly as before, you may worry that you are headed to divorce court. Instead, it could be that your partner has been losing the main brain chemical (or neurotransmitter) that supports human connection and emotional engagement.

Much of what you are going to find in this book is related to helping you recognize and respond to how Parkinson's changes the way that your partner can express love and connection. I hope that understanding more about these effects will make it possible for you to see more clearly how PD is affecting your partner, affecting your relationship, and affecting you.

It has been my experience that most online sources and books on Parkinson's will not tell you enough about this aspect of Parkinson's. Many only devote a page or two to the issues, concerns, and needs of the PWP's partner or spouse. In the same way, your partner's medical providers are also unlikely to say much to you about how your PWP's condition will impact your day-to-day life. And that's too bad.

Amid the bad luck of developing Parkinson's Disease, it is incredibly good luck when a PWP has a committed partner, someone to walk alongside them throughout the long course of this disease. It's a sad reality that there is no cure for Parkinson's, and in almost every case there is no stopping the slow and then faster decline of this condition. A loving and committed partner makes a big difference in the quality of life for a PWP.

So why do the books stay silent? Why does the doctor almost ignore you? It seems neurologists and Movement Disorders Specialists in the US study very little about the role a partner can play in the well-being of a PWP. They are not specialists in family dynamics or the day-to-day strain of living with Parkinson's, so they can't say much to you or to your partner about these aspects of the disease.

That is why I've written this book. I lived with and loved my husband, Peter, for the last eight years of his life. He'd had Parkinson's for fourteen years when I met him and for nearly twenty-three years when he died. Along the way, I learned a lot, starting with what I heard from a local Movement Disorders Specialist who took the time to teach me to care for Peter.

I've also been an active participant in several online spaces where the wives, partners, and caregivers of people with Parkinson's join each other in the virtual world, to vent, to learn, to celebrate, and to grieve. The people, mostly women, in these online groups and forums have created a no-judgment zone in which the strains of loving, caring for, and losing a partner with Parkinson's make sense.

It still makes me a little crazy that in all of my years of caring for my husband, only one medical person, an advanced trainee in geriatrics, looked directly at me to say, "You are doing a really good job." I still feel myself tearing up at how much this meant to me and how much I needed to hear those words—how much I needed to be seen.

So I am here to tell you, "You, too, are doing a good job." How do I know that? Because you've opened this book to learn about how to take care of your partner *and* yourself.

Why? Because I know that you are part of your partner's struggle to hold on to his sense of well-being, his humanity, and his sense of himself. I know this, too, because you've taken this step to really face the hard truths of living with and loving a person with Parkinson's.

A caution before we dive in. **Please do not share this book with your partner.** There are many good books, websites, and other ways to share information with your PWP. I describe three good ones in Appendix 1. This book talks about the challenges of being a CP, a Caregiving Partner, and these are things that you need to be aware of that might be completely overwhelming for them to think about. This is not meant to keep secrets from your partner but to shield them from too quickly having to realize how PD will change their day-to-day life and from having to recognize just how hard you will have to work to protect the two of you and your partnership.

Another note. I'm writing this book for any committed partner of a person with Parkinson's. While the gender of the person who is walking alongside a person with PD tells us nothing about what that person will need, there are twice as many men as women with PD. That is why for some instances in this book I will refer to the person with PD as "he." And, because the partners I've known and learned from have mostly been women, I often refer to the partner as "she." To be sure, Parkinson's is diagnosed in people of every gender and orientation, and the lucky ones have a person—a spouse, a partner, a significant other or chosen family member willing to walk this path with them. And you may not be your PWP's partner. While I've written this book for a spouse or partner of a person with Parkinson's, you may be a child or grandchild, a parent, or a friend to someone with Parkinson's. If so, I hope that you will find information here to help you understand and support your PWP, whatever your connection with them. So whoever you are, please know that this book is written for you, as you recognize the commitment you have made to a person diagnosed with PD.

Third, to dive into this book, you are going to put on what you may have heard described as your "big girl panties." It's a silly expression, but it means standing up to hard truths as they come along and taking care of business. There is no way around it. Parkinson's is hard. But then again, if you live long enough, *something* in your life is going to be hard.

I don't think there is any point in comparing one disease, disorder, injury, or family difficulty against another. It is enough to say that Parkinson's is the one you've decided to read about now, and I am going to try to tell you what I have learned from my own experiences—from in-person conversations, blog posts, social media, and other places—about this Parkinson's experience.

People sometimes talk about the Parkinson's journey, but this really isn't a trip anyone wants to take. I think living with a partner with PD is like waking up and finding that the familiar ground all around you is starting to get wetter, softer, and muddier. Unfamiliar vegetation is sprouting up at your feet. Lots of weeds are showing up with an occasional blossom or two as well. It's getting much harder for the two of you to manage. Gusts of wind keep pushing you off course, and over time, you—the partner—must be the one who keeps the two of you from being blown to the muddy ground.

At some point, someone will respond to learning about your partner's PD by saying, "Take care of yourself. " They probably mean well, but don't actually offer much to help improve anything. Most of us want to respond (but rarely say aloud), "How on earth do I do that?" I hope that this book will give you answers to that very question.

I wrote the book to give you information, ideas, skills, techniques, and other tidbits related to being in a partnership when PD is part of the picture. You'll find things I wish I could have found when I met and married Peter, knowing he had PD but really having no idea of what might lie ahead. (Nor did he because we were each living that *it's just about the movement* illusion at the time.) You won't find much about the medical aspects of PD, or medications, or about managing the physical aspects of PD. There are so many wonderful and well-researched resources around to help you navigate those issues. And, as specific symptoms come up in our conversation, you may want to consult one of the medically oriented books or online sources mentioned in Appendix 1.

I want to do something different here. I want to help you think about what your partner's PD means for your partnership and for you as an individual.

So, I am glad you are here. Not glad that you are facing Parkinson's with someone who is in your life, but glad that your partner has you and glad to offer you whatever wisdom I can. I hope this book helps you to be more prepared and to have more tools and strategies to sustain yourself and your relationship as you stand beside your Person through this experience.

In Part One I'll help you make a mental reset so that you understand why it is so important to know that the changes of PD take place in the brain and profoundly impact the way it interacts with the body. I'll discuss some of the supports that you'll want to have in place to get started building a PD life that cares for your Person and for you.

If you are mainly looking for information about Parkinson's itself, look in the Appendix to find some of the many resources I found useful: books, websites, online forums, and community resources.

Then, on to the main purpose of this book—to understand how PD impacts the person as a partner. In Part Two, I focus on the many ways that Parkinson's might affect your life together. You will be able to consider adaptations and adjustments and to work on short check-in exercises after each chapter that will help you, in your own right and as part of a couple, to sustain a loving and dignified relationship alongside your Partner with Parkinson's, your PWP.

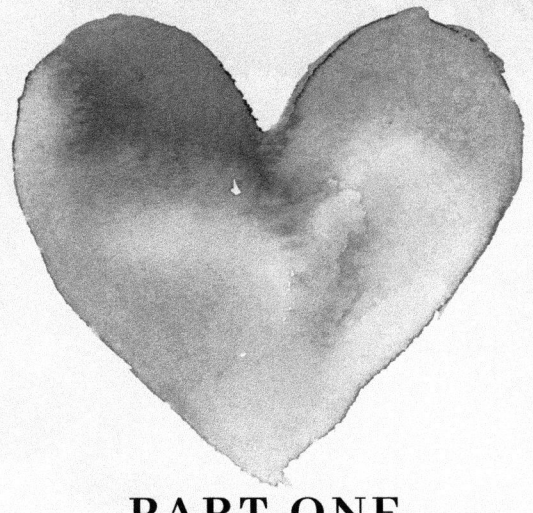

PART ONE

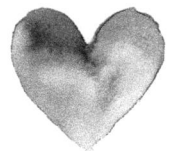

CHAPTER ONE

Not Just the Muscles

To begin, I want you to know that Parkinson's is not just a disease of the muscles and movement. It's not surprising that you might think it is, since for many years after 1871, when James Parkinson noticed several patients who all had similar symptoms of stiffness, stooping shoulders, and shaky muscles and called it "the shaking palsy," it seemed that only the muscular and movement systems of the body were affected by this widespread disease. Today, it is well known that there is more to Parkinson's than problems with how the body moves and stands, and that Parkinson's affects both the body and the mind.

Mostly, Parkinson's is a disease of the brain. However, it is not just the tissues of the brain that change with it. Parkinson's affects the brain chemicals that send messages from one part of the brain to many other parts and that spark the signals directing the body, mind, emotions, and intellect. Those chemical changes don't show up in pictures. Just as you can't use an X-ray to detect a fever, a brain scan won't give the final answer when Parkinson's is suspected.

Partners of People with Parkinson's often get confused because there are so many things besides movement that break down as the disease progresses. Very often, partners will ask about puzzling changes that they have observed. They ask, "My partner has had a real change of personality, has a lot of pain, craves sweets, or spends money and gambles without considering the consequences" (among other manifestations). Then they ask, "Is that unusual?" And while a doctor may say such manifestations are unusual, very often in the online communities, people experiencing the day-to-day of a Parkinson's life will comment, "May be unusual. But I've seen that too."

If your experience is like those I've read and heard about in my online and in-person conversations with other PD partners, your doctors have said little to you about how PD will change the PWP. Whether it is because the doctors do not want to alarm their patient with the enormity of a new diagnosis or because these couple-level issues are outside of their awareness, it seems doctors do not educate PWPs and their partners about the kinds of experiences, interactions, and changes that are quite common in the lives of people who have Parkinson's.

Even books that focus on the day-to-day management of the disease do not seem to give you much guidance on how to recognize, respond, adapt, and manage as Parkinson's changes your spouse. The regular doctor's visits that are usual in PD care never really seem to have a space to ask about how the couple is managing. Many caregivers tell us it feels as if they are complaining or that they will be seen as unwilling caregivers if they raise these issues. Interestingly, it seems that even a Movement Disorders Specialist, who offers a more expert approach to PD management than a general neurologist, may not pay much attention to these complexities.

The Couple-level Impact of Parkinson's Disease

It is the lucky person with Parkinson's who has a spouse or partner in their corner. Even though the medical profession seems not to make good use of this fact, the partner often forms an essential part of the ongoing care for a person diagnosed with PD. As things progress, partners take on more caregiving responsibilities, and the relationship shifts. As this happens, partners can feel as if they are an invisible person in the background.

HIPAA (the Health Insurance Portability and Accountability Act) requires US medical providers to hold medical communication and information private unless they have been specifically given permission by the patient.

With PD, this devotion to patient privacy may prevent vital conversations between the PD physician and the partner from happening during the stages when preventive measures can increase the person's ability to manage as the disease advances. Even though you may be highly interested in being a support to your partner, you can remain excluded from important discussions in the earliest stages after the diagnosis.

Too often, caregivers find that they have to jump in midstream. Compounding this, if your habits, cultural, or religious values make you prefer to let your husband lead, then you wait for permission to be involved in and informed about his care. All of this means that your feelings of invisibility and unimportance can come from a real place. As a caregiver, it all compounds your stress and anxiety.

Paying attention to the couple-level impact of Parkinson's helps you identify the range of changes in your life and can help you make decisions about where and how you need to ask for help, to make changes, or to change your expectation to maintain a positive life in the face of the changes to come. You can ask yourself what has changed in your interpersonal life—your partnership with your PWP. Other changes can be physical—your partner may not be able to carry out physical chores, help to maintain your home, or contribute to their own or your economic and spiritual well-being. The questions at the end of this chapter can help you think about what you are seeing as Parkinson's affects you and your partner.

It might be easier not to pay attention to these questions. However, I think that noticing what is going on, and even writing down the things that you are seeing, doesn't make them any worse. And as you pay attention to what is happening, you have more of a chance to make informed decisions about what you, your partner, and others need.

Check-in for Chapter One

Think of this first check-in as a kind of status report. Read each item in the chart. Ask yourself, "How are you doing? Where are things today?" Briefly describe the changes you have noticed since PD entered your lives. At the end of each section, use the blank lines to add in other items in that category that are specific to your situation.

Don't let this process overwhelm you. Just make quick notes to yourself, making sure that you focus first on yourself. Then turn your attention to your Partner with Parkinson's. How is he or she doing?

Working in this order may be unfamiliar and even uncomfortable. After all, most of us feel that once our partner is being affected by PD, our first responsibility is to them rather than ourselves.

I'm sure that you won't lose track of the chance to think about your partner, so I want to be sure that you think about you. Start there because noticing how things are with you helps to make sure that your PWP has a well-functioning caregiver. But these questions are also important because you are a whole person and are entitled to pay attention to your own wants and needs.

Relationships

Briefly describe the status of each relationship. Has PD changed them?

☐ PWP   ☐ Children/Grandchildren

☐ Parents   ☐ Other family

☐ Friends   ☐ Community

☐ Work/professional colleagues

Now for your PWP. Based on your own observations, how are these relationships for them?

- ☐ PWP
- ☐ Parents
- ☐ Friends
- ☐ Work/professional colleagues
- ☐ Children/Grandchildren
- ☐ Other family
- ☐ Community

Practical Things

How are these practical aspects of daily life today?

- ☐ Daily cleaning and maintenance
- ☐ House and yard maintenance
- ☐ Moving to a new home
- ☐ Income and money management
- ☐ Adapting your home/safety and fall prevention
- ☐ Food shopping and meal preparation

What do you notice about these practical things in your PWP's daily life?

- ☐ Daily cleaning and maintenance
- ☐ House and yard maintenance
- ☐ Moving to a new home
- ☐ Income and money management
- ☐ Adapting your home/safety and fall prevention
- ☐ Food shopping and meal preparation

Life Course

How is the course of your life?

- ☐ Job and career path
- ☐ Retirement
- ☐ Education and Training
- ☐ Economic well-being

And now your PWP's life course. How are things?

- ☐ Job and career path
- ☐ Retirement
- ☐ Education and Training
- ☐ Economic well-being

Self-care and Spirit

How is your overall well-being?

☐ Sobriety and recovery   ☐ Exercise and sports

☐ Vacation and travel   ☐ Creative activities and hobbies

☐ Religious observances & obligations   ☐ Attendance at religious services/events

☐ Changed relationship with God

And how is your PWP's overall well-being?

☐ Sobriety and recovery   ☐ Exercise and sports

☐ Vacation and travel   ☐ Creative activities and hobbies

☐ Religious observances & obligations   ☐ Attendance at religious services/events

☐ Changed relationship with God

Health

How is your health?

☐ Your own physical health   ☐ Your own physical health

☐ Health of children, parents, others   ☐ Your own mental health

☐ Your PWP's mental health   ☐ Mental health of others

Apart from PD itself, how are your partner's mental and physical health?

☐ Your PWP's physical health

☐ Your PWP's mental health

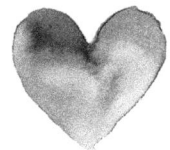

CHAPTER TWO

Resources for the Journey Ahead

I think it helps to be as clear-eyed as we can be when bracing ourselves to face a challenging life situation. Getting ready in this way is an important part of becoming a partner to someone who has PD.

Yes, there is also a place for holding on to hope, which helps us to continue over the long haul. However, in my view, it is even more important for your longevity to have a practical and realistic assessment of your resources, your needs, and your relationship.

Respect Your Own Reaction

Of course, the person who has been diagnosed with Parkinson's Disease is most directly affected by the news that he or she has acquired what my PWP husband called a "progressive, incurable disease." The feelings of the person with this tough diagnosis are of prime importance, and that is as it should be. However, this book gives you, the Parkinson's partner, the chance to pay attention to *your* feelings and reactions.

You likely have both noticed problems with movement, mood, energy, or motivation that prompted you to see a doctor. Sometimes, these changes lead to a diagnosis right away, Still, it's common for this process to have taken months or even years. Whatever your partner's response to the diagnosis, and no matter how hard you are working to support them, you also have your own reaction. You may feel afraid, or maybe it's a relief to have a clear diagnosis. Some partners feel comforted when they hear that carbidopa/levodopa (trade name Sinemet™), a "gold standard" medication, will probably help. However, along with that sense of relief can come deep disappointment that a chronic and unrelenting illness has entered your lives.

You probably will not tell many people about feeling this way, but you can be sure that there is no shame in experiencing such normal human emotions. You would have to be a robot, a pathological person, or a saint to have no feelings at all about the losses and disappointment to come. Being aware of your own point of view—your own reaction—is important to help your partner *and* to help you. Become familiar with the full range of experience that arise with this news. I believe an important policy is this one: "No shame here."

A Focus on the Future

I live in Maine, in a house built more than 160 years ago by a ship's carpenter. In those days, every sailing vessel's crew included a carpenter because there were always things that would break and need fixing during a voyage. Still, the sailors would say that they did not want to build the boat as they were sailing it. In the same way, you don't want to wait until a new problem related to PD arises to start learning what you need to know. One of my goals in writing this book is to help you get ready with what you will need to know and what you might need to do as Parkinson's Disease progresses. By doing this, I hope to help you maintain a sense of dignity and love in your relationship.

Parkinson's is a one-way road. There are not, as I'm writing this, any known cures for PD. Yes, there are new advances in brain surgery for PD such as various forms of deep brain stimulation, and new medications are under development. And from time to time, you'll read about new research findings. However, there is no treatment so far that can reverse the course of PD.

Being realistic, you understand that PD will be a lifelong presence in your PWP's life, and in yours, for as long as you are together.

There can be unrecognized changes to the person's brain long before the major physical symptoms lead to a diagnosis of Parkinson's. And since these changes can affect the ability to focus, to make plans and carry them out, you are likely to play an increasing role in organizing and planning your partner's care.

Your partner may not recognize these changes right away, and you will have to decide whether or not to bring up with your partner the ways that he or she is becoming less organized and effective. Research[1] shows that Parkinson's will reduce the person's ability to actively participate in this kind of planning and organization. Ideally, you can jointly plan how you can work together. Still, be prepared to have to take the lead as time passes in planning for his or her Parkinson's care, as well as in other aspects of your life together. In Part II, I'll discuss more about these and other adjustments to your partnership that you can expect to make.

First People to Help: Movement Disorders Specialists (MDS) and Elder Law Attorneys

After a person is diagnosed with PD, there are two things that can be taken care of in the early months. Establish a relationship with a Movement Disorders Specialist, a neurologist who has additional specialized training in managing Parkinson's, and with an attorney who works across many areas of practice to protect the rights, finances, and well-being of older people and those with disabilities.

---

1 https://www.ncbi.nlm.nih.gov/pmc/articles/PMC3171949/shows

Movement Disorders Specialist

A diagnosis of Parkinson's may come from a person's primary care provider, or a general neurologist. Even though Parkinson's looks vastly different from one person to another, the classic signs are remarkably similar to the things James Parkinson saw over 200 years ago. Sometimes a primary care doctor may start a person on carbidopa/levodopa right away, even before making the referral to a neurologist.

Whatever your doctor decides, experienced PD partners suggest that instead of a general neurologist, it is worthwhile to seek a Movement Disorders Specialist from the start. The Movement Disorder specialty is a relatively new one, and in some areas, there are not as many of these well-trained doctors as are needed.[2]

In our state there were very few Parkinson's specialty doctors, and after we arrived here, it took a long time to get a first appointment with an MDS. For a while, we had to drive a few hours out of state for my husband to have well-trained providers. Even if it is quite a trip to get there, even if you are not sure that you will need one, try right away to set an appointment. The MDS neurologist has received advanced training, and even done research, on the specific needs of patients who have Parkinson's and related movement disorders. Unlike community neurologists, who need to address a wide range of problems of the brain and spinal cord, the MDS has a more focused practice and more expertise.

When you make this appointment, it can help if you also start to have practical conversations with your partner right away about involving you in his medical visits. It may worry your partner to think that someday they may need this kind of help, but still, the time will come when you need to help with communicating with the doctor. It's beneficial to have already built a relationship with the MDS.

---

2 The International Parkinson and Movement Disorder Society has an online directory of these specialists. https://mds.movementdisorders.org/directory/. The Parkinson's Foundation's Helpline can also help with finding a Movement Disorders Specialist Helpline 1.800.4PD.INFO (473-4636)

Once you begin to work with MDS doctors, you might find nurse practitioners and physician's assistants working with your doctor. When you are getting acquainted with your partner's new MDS, ask the doctor if he or she coordinates care with one of these physician extenders. That way you won't be surprised if on future visits the person who comes into the room first is not the doctor you met.

As I mentioned earlier, the medical privacy laws in the US stop doctors from communicating with you about your PD partner. But you can still communicate with the doctor without permission. Some CPs send an email message, or a written note, or fax their partners' doctors before the appointment, to make sure that the doctor is working with the information he or she needs to best care for their patient. And once you've met with an Elder Law attorney, you will be able to have Medical Power of Attorney, which allows two-way communication with your partner's doctors.

When the MDS watches how PD is changing a person's physical status, he or she should also watch for cognitive and emotional changes. While this doctor may track and document these changes, they are unlikely to address the impact that these symptoms have on your day-to-day life at home and your capacity as a caregiver. That is why I encourage you to be proactive in planning for your future Parkinson's Life.

Elder Law Attorney

In the online PD communities, it's common for new PD caregivers to get the advice to secure their financial future right away. This advice may sound greedy or insensitive, but—in the United States especially—this is critical since the spotty network of publicly supported care (primarily Medicaid and Medicare) leaves many individuals and families struggling to manage.

That is why the first piece of advice many caregivers hear online is to see one of these specialized attorneys. While most lawyers focus on one specific area of the law, such as taxes, estates, criminal law, or real estate, these lawyers focus their practice on the full range of legal needs that arise as people age, needs that are also relevant for people of all ages living with a disability.

Parkinson's can be a costly disease. Getting help to pay for these costs is a complicated issue. Some people have long-term care insurance, which can be used to pay for in-home care or care in a facility, but such policies are expensive and may be hard to get after a person has been diagnosed with PD. It is important at the start to get the advice of this kind of attorney. Their knowledge of how the laws of Medicaid and Medicare and how the trusts, estate, and insurance laws in your state operate can make a real difference, both in your ability to have the money, the information, and the legal rights you need to care for your PWP and to care for yourself.

But what is the rush? If Parkinson's is a slowly progressing illness, then isn't it early and even a little ghoulish, to think in those terms—long-term care, estate planning—right away? Perhaps, but know that there is at least one provision in the Medicaid law that requires a five-year waiting period before you can benefit. Many people are surprised to learn that Medicare, which supports medical treatment for older Americans, does not pay for long-term care. And, Medicaid, the United States' public funding plan for the disabled and elderly, does not allow a person to own more than a minimal amount to be eligible for this financial help. The rules around qualifying for help to pay for the care of a person with a disabling condition are complicated—and they vary from state to state.

You might think that when the time comes, you could just transfer your car or house, your boat or bank accounts into your own name. However, here is where Medicaid's "five-year look-back" comes up. Unless you follow them carefully, the Medicaid rules could make you wait five years after making this kind of transfer before they will help to fund the person's care. Talking to an Elder Law Attorney early gives you the best chance of making the financial decisions that will give you the most control over how you and your partner will manage.

You may think that you don't have enough to need this kind of professional help—and attorney fees can be steep. Still, many times an initial consultation is free and may be enough to guide you to take a lot of important early steps on your own. In fact, people who have a lot of assets—money, stocks, businesses, or property—have more flexibility if they make a mistake in these early weeks of adjusting and planning. If you don't have as much to work with, then you will benefit by getting this guidance within a few months of the diagnosis. Find an Elder Law Attorney in your area online using the National Academy of Elder Law Attorneys (naela.org/findlawyer) to help you.

It's also important to know that some families wait too long to take this important step. Your PWP will need to be legally capable of signing POA and other documents that your Elder Law Attorney develops with you. If you wait, the person with Parkinson's may lose their capacity to make these decisions. An early visit to the Elder Law Attorney is a way of making sure that you have these documents available when and if they become necessary.

My husband was a lawyer and paid close attention to these things. Peter knew he had PD and he had the documents drawn up to be sure that, when the time came, I could receive and deposit his pension checks and pay the bills. Then we didn't even think about the documents for years. Later, when it was time, there was no question that I could handle our household finances. If you get these things in place, then you can "set it and forget it."

Other Resources

For many couples, the Elder Law Attorney and MDS will be the principal professional supporters. The demands on you can be relatively few in the early stages of caregiving. However, this isn't always the case. PD may have been quietly depleting the dopamine stores in the PWP's brain for many years, so that by the time the symptoms become bothersome enough to see a doctor, the PD is already fairly far advanced.

You'll want to know that your partner's primary care provider has experience with PWPs and will help you both to coordinate care with the MDS and other specialists. It's useful to gather information from each of a PWP's medical providers and to understand their roles. The time may come when you will have to coordinate decisions about medications, therapies, hospitalizations, and other processes. You will want to know that your various medical providers can be and are willing to be in touch with each other and that they will welcome you as a part of your partner's care. After all, you will at some point become the team leader and quarterback of this team of providers. Start scouting now.

Along with setting up these connections for legal and medical help, it can be useful to search for other information to plan for your future. Sometimes in the wake of a diagnosis of PD, a couple can plan to build a dream home in a community where they hope to live comfortably. This can be the opportunity to find a home that will be accessible and safe for you and your PWP. Also keep in mind that as the person's needs change, there may be more frequent medical visits. You may want to use in-home caregivers who live nearby and might even choose an out-of-home facility.

Many times, a caregiver will make a heartfelt promise to her partner to "never put you in a home." This is an easy and natural promise to make, but it is not always the right promise, and it can sometimes be hard to keep. Some caregivers exhaust themselves and become less effective simply to maintain this promise. Not only that, insisting on doing all the caregiving yourself keeps you both from having the supportive care that a well-chosen residential PD setting can provide. Finding extra care with managing the symptoms of PD, at home or in a facility, will free you to be friends, partners, and even lovers again.

Build an Exercise Program

My husband, Peter, was a lifelong athlete. He'd been a varsity runner in college (and was very proud of his record of a 4-minute, 13-second mile). Later in life, he enjoyed a variety of sports, and we both believed that the habits of regular exercise helped slow the progression of his PD for many years. He enjoyed using a specialized stationary bike (Theracycle. com) and rode it daily. For years, I slept in most mornings and woke to the sound of his cycling away, his effort boosted by the bike's motor. Exercise is known to help PWPs sustain balance, guard against falls, and build overall wellness. There is even evidence that some kinds of exercise programs can slow the progression of PD.[3]

Developing a habit of regular exercise may require you to be the cheerleader if your PWP is not enthusiastic about it. Whether your partner chooses biking, Rock Steady Boxing (rocksteadyboxing.org), Tai Chi, or just regular walking, you can join in with them.

In fact, exercise is so critical for continued wellbeing that one expert (Friedman, 2013) gives caregivers full permission to nag about exercise (and only about exercise, he says)!

Maintaining Relationships

Along with building these professional resources, you will want to set the stage early on to maintain your connections to friends, family, and your community. Do you have a spiritual practice, a faith community where you find companions and practice your religion? Some people have found that their religious communities have engaged readily and happily to help, while letting the PWP and the PD Caregiver set the tone, timing, and direction of that help. Others, sadly, tell us that as the couple turned inward to focus on the increasing care needs of a PWP, friends and the

---

3 https://www.medicalnewstoday.com/articles/parkinsons-disease-move-regularly-with-intensity-to-delay-symptoms

religious community faded away. Maybe they fade away because they do not know whether, how, or how often to help. They may not know what's useful, or even fear they might be drawn too firmly or too permanently into the day-to-day-ness of Parkinson's.

Then too, sometimes unexpected people may say they find it hard to see the losses your PWP is undergoing. Still, the kind of comment that starts, "It's too hard for me to see him like that," must be one of the most selfish statements that could be made to a couple in the weeds of the ongoing, unrelenting losses PD brings. The statement does not convey tenderheartedness or sensitivity, but a kind of self-absorption that can break a caregiver's heart.

Don't wait for something like this to happen. Instead, let your faith community know that you welcome their help and ask them if you may reach out, even if it becomes too difficult to bring your PWP to participate in religious practices in person. Similarly, reach out to friends and family, letting them know that while you are managing at the present, you may want and need their help in some way in the future. Asking for this kind of commitment early on may help you to maintain a connection with people who will become a lifeline for you and your PWP.

Your Internal Resources

Being a Parkinson's caregiver isn't easy. You will need patience, a willingness to let the person with PD take the lead in his or her care, and the ability to stand by—ready to jump in when your help is needed. You may notice that your partner begins to "drop the ball" as he or she agrees to plans and fails to carry them out or forgets them altogether. It must be very unnerving to a person who has been a well-functioning adult to recognize that things have started to slip. Whether you talk directly to your PWP about these changes or not, you'll need to be alert to them yourself.

I think things can work well when the caregiver is able to stand to the side, to supplement what the PWP can do for themselves, to take over when that is needed, and to wait when it isn't. Early on, you'll help your partner by identifying the team members that I've described—the doctors, lawyers, and community resources that you can turn to when you need them. You can contribute to getting your finances set, establishing and maintaining lines of communication with medical providers, and helping your partner to establish a regular program of exercise.

At the same time, many caregivers have a very busy personal and working life of their own, one that may end up taking a back seat to the demands of Parkinson's. Your internal resources are just important as the external ones we've been discussing. Apart from your paid employment, your usual activities are going to be impacted by caregiving.

Hold On to Who You Are

"I know I am not supposed to want anything. But I feel so sad and worn out." In just a few words, this young woman, who was caring for a grandparent with Parkinson's, revealed the sorrow and despair that had filled her daily life. Somehow, there are many caregivers who have the idea that depriving themselves goes with the decision to take care of a PWP. This misunderstanding seems to shape the daily lives of many caregivers, draining color and warmth from a relationship.

Your distress does not improve your PWP's life. Instead of immediately stepping away from hobbies and activities, something as small as a short walk, spending half an hour on a small aspect of one a hobby, or just taking a breath of fresh air, can keep your *self* in the picture.

Taking care of yourself is part of taking the long view of the new kind of relationship that comes from being a caregiver. Before you completely give up things that are important to you, step back without stepping away.

Are you a member of a community organization—a chorus, a Girl Scout or Campfire leader? Do you have a volunteer job? Are there specific things at home that give you great satisfaction? These activities are part of your sense of self—of your identity—and it's important to include them in your audit/survey of your caregiving resources.

It is easy for caregivers to lose sight of these parts of themselves as they become immersed in the demands of daily care. Holding on to your own identity as a worker, person of faith, volunteer, and/or family member is a tool for sustaining your caregiving self. In Chapter Six, there will be more to read about refreshing yourself as you go. Throughout all of this, remember you are important, and *your* needs count too.

Your capacity to earn in paid employment or in a business is an important support for you, for your family, and for the PWP. As you first walk alongside your PWP as a care partner, you may not notice many differences in how your partner's PD affects your working life. Later, however, you may reach a point where balancing your job and your role as a care partner or caregiver will affect your relationship to your paid work.

Think carefully about when you decide to inform your employer that your partner has been diagnosed with PD. Being intentional about what you say early on may allow you more latitude in job placement and promotion opportunities. Of course you don't plan to lie, but volunteering the information in casual conversations may cause it to affect decisions about placement and promotion. You want to maintain control of the information. Keeping the diagnosis separate from your workplace conversations may be a good idea.[4]

Some caregivers have had wonderful experiences with their workplaces and felt supported when they needed flexibility, or even time off, to care for a family member. However, because the FMLA (Family and Medical Leave Act)[5] can be complex, it may be useful to think about how your workplace accommodates workers' disabilities, and then research the company's policies before deciding whether and when to talk about your partner's diagnosis.

---

4 https://www.apdaparkinson.org/article/when-to-disclose-parkinsons/

5 https://www.aplaceformom.com/caregiver-resources/articles/fmla-facts

Discussing PD

When did you learn about your partner's PD diagnosis? Sometimes, partners go through the process of diagnosis together, but other times, a person may learn on their own about having PD and then will decide about when and how to talk about this diagnosis with you. It is very personal news. I think that knowing about the PD diagnosis from the start makes it easier to learn together how you will integrate your partner's new situation into your relationship.

If your PWP assumes that you are automatically going to act as care partner and caregiver for them, then you have a right to be well informed about this condition. If they choose to keep their PD diagnosis or what they learn in meetings with their doctor private, then how can you participate in their care? I believe that you need to know enough about your partner's medical care to be able to be a competent caregiver.

Talk together about what you each want. Your life has been altered by this information. What can you each do? What do you each expect? It is hard to know at the beginning what specific changes will come. But you can set the stage for a healthy partnership by focusing on what you each want, what your worries are, and how you hope to navigate this new future together.

What if your partner won't discuss PD? Some people shy away from talking about difficult things. Sometimes, this reluctance stems from the way the person was raised. Family and culture have a strong impact on what we see as unmentionable. So sometimes a PWP does not have much awareness of his or her own feelings about this new reality. Still other situations can involve a PWP who does not feel that he owes a partner answers or explanations and just expects her to perform her duties to home and family with few questions.

Certainly, there is no one right way to be a family and no one right way to build a caregiving partnership. Whatever your family's style of communication, be sure a decision not to talk about these issues is just that—a decision and not simply something that gets put off until later. Think about how your family has handled difficulties in the past and ask yourself what you hope for. You'll need a clear-eyed view of this new situation as you start to gather the resources you will need to build as you face this challenge.

You and your PWP will also want to think about how to talk to family members and close friends. Think through what you want to say and what you want to hear from your family as your time with PD goes along. You don't have to pass on every detail about your partner's medical condition to let these important people know that there has been a change, and there will be challenges to come.

I think it is a mistake to deflect questions when friends and family ask about your partner's well-being. Often, caregivers will only say that their partner is "fine" or "doing well," even as the symptoms of PD are progressing, and the caregiving is becoming more challenging. It may be wiser to let at least a few people know about how things really are. For instance, you might say, "He's getting used to the way PD is changing him." It's an accurate statement. It's optimistic, but also gives people a heads-up that things are not the same. And, when you respond to these questions, make sure you include yourself. Saying something like, "So far I've been able to do what he needs, for now," lets people know, discreetly, that you are having to put in effort to help take care of your PWP.

Parkinson's Is Forever

This hard truth, that there is no cure for Parkinson's Disease, is one we caregivers share with many families in which someone has a permanent condition. Whether from an illness like FDR's polio, an injury like *Superman* actor Christopher Reeve's quadriplegia, or Parkinson's, many families face their futures knowing an illness or disability will be part of their lives. This means that the planning and thinking that this book guides you towards can serve you for the rest of your marriage, for the rest of your lives together.

The promise of "a cure in ten years" has been repeated for years, and despite advances in understanding how the progressive loss of dopamine affects the brain and body, we still do not have a cure. Fortunately, the "gold standard" medication, carbidopa/levodopa, offers symptom relief to many people with Parkinson's. In the brain, levodopa is turned into dopamine, while carbidopa helps reduce some of the negative side effects of having dopamine in the digestive system. Other medications are available as well.[6] Your Movement Disorders Specialist is responsible for choosing, prescribing, and adjusting Parkinson's medications. And while these medications don't completely interrupt the symptoms of Parkinson's disease, along with exercise, they do offer many PWPs the chance to continue with their daily life for years, and even decades. Even the newest research on using stem cells to treat Parkinson's[7] only aims to treat symptoms, without halting the progression of the disease.

The day may come when newer interventions, like deep brain stimulation or other medications, will make Parkinson's a thing of the past. For now, it is important to watch out for the charlatans who offer false information and the online or print writers who mislead worried and desperate Parkinson's patients and their families by reporting a small discovery about one PD-like symptom in mice as though it offers an imminent cure. This kind of cruelty absorbs too much mental and emotional energy and offers a kind of false hope. I believe that it's possible to lose precious years chasing a cure that hasn't yet been found.

I look forward to the day when this book becomes obsolete. Until then, please don't chase false promises. At the time I am writing this (2022), there is no cure, no diet, supplements, or stem-cell treatment that is known to cure PD. The most effective interventions are exercise, prescription medications like carbidopa/levodopa to control symptoms, and deep-brain stimulation to reduce tremors.

---

6 An excellent online guide to Parkinson's Medications is available here https://davisphinneyfoundation.org/medication-guide/

7 https://www.nature.com/articles/d41586-021-02622-3

The false promises of a cure for Parkinson's can make us lose sight of the value of careful treatment with the current array of medications and interventions. While the pace of developing new medications has been frustratingly slow, research has given us a lot more information about the physical and psychological characteristics of Parkinson's. As PD researchers and people with Parkinson's learned more about how to manage the physical symptoms, the stiffness and shakiness that are the hallmarks of the disease, it began to be clear that there are other equally common characteristics that affect the quality of life for people with Parkinson's Disease and their family members.

A difficult but important realization about PD caregiving comes as you understand that your path and your partner's will diverge as the disease progresses. However close you have been, you will realize that only one of you is going through the experience of having PD. You, the caregiver, can walk closely beside your partner, but the challenges that you and they face are different.

In the remaining chapters of *Love, Dignity, and Parkinson's* I will focus on your role as caregiver and the important things you can do to sustain the two of you as you travel these parallel but different paths.

Check in for Chapter Two

This chapter has set the stage for you to look at the initial resources that are necessary to virtually every PD caregiver. This check-in will give you a sense of where you might start to gather these essential assets as you move through life with Parkinson's.

- What preparations have you and your PWP made for changes to come?
- Are there other preparations you'd like to make? How can you start?
- How easy is it for you and your PWP to communicate?
- If it is not easy, will you be able to improve communication with your PWP? How will you start?
- How have you begun to build the resources to sustain you as a caregiver?
- Where are you making room in your current social networks for the ways PD may change you?
- What might you do now to make it easier to reach out to others for help as the need arises?
- How else can you pave the way for an easier time in the future?

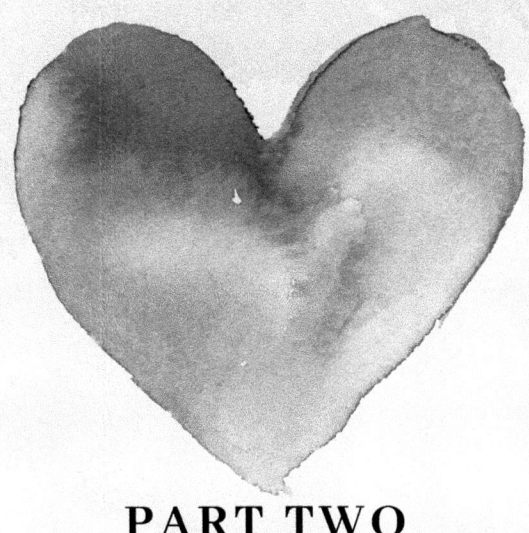

PART TWO

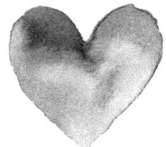

CHAPTER THREE

Parkinson's, the Thief

Parkinson's affects the levels of dopamine in the brain and in the body. This neurotransmitter is a messenger chemical that affects many different functions. As dopamine levels in the person's brain decrease, there are effects that, though less visible than the changes in posture, gait, and balance, present the greatest challenges for the caregiver-PWP relationship. These are sometimes referred to as non-motor effects, to distinguish them from the movement-related features of PD. Parkinson's non-motor effects impact the PWP's presence, engagement, stamina, and well-being, which in turn can affect the caregiving spouse's ability to support the PWP.

Dopamine—a Brain Chemical with Many Functions

The changes that PD couples face are often linked to the non-motor aspects of PD, but all symptoms of PD (both the movement and muscle symptoms and the non-motor effects) show the many ways in which the body changes as dopamine levels decrease in the brain.

Dopamine is a substance that occurs naturally—primarily in the brain, but in other parts of the body as well. It is called a neurotransmitter because it does the important job of sending signals between neurons. You can think of dopamine molecules as messengers that travel many routes, sending messages to different parts of the brain. The main thing for PD caregivers to know is that Parkinson's Disease symptoms (the tremor, stiffness, and changes in behavior, empathy, learning, thinking, emotions, and relating) come about because the full amount of dopamine isn't available in the brain.

People who are eventually diagnosed with PD have been losing dopamine for some time, in some cases for years. Maybe, in the future, doctors will know to look for the behavioral and emotional signs of PD even before the muscle stiffness, halting gait, and tremor show themselves. We can hope that with earlier recognition, interventions can be made available during the initial stages of PD.

The patterns of PD, and the way dopamine depletion affects an individual, vary so much that it is hard for even the best specialists to predict the ways in which PD will affect an individual person's life. The truism "if you've seen one person with Parkinson's, you've seen one person with Parkinson's" applies.

For couples and caregivers, it is important to know that many of the challenges PD couples face are related to these non-motor aspects. Sadly, too often doctors, both primary care doctors, neurologists, and even Movement Disorders Specialists, do not point to these early non-motor symptoms. Caregivers discover that these changes may be due to Parkinson's somewhat farther along.

When doctors and scientists do talk about the cognitive changes of PD, they separate out the various brain functions and talk about them one at time. These discussions may be scientifically precise, but they do not do a good job of reflecting the way that Parkinson's can challenge partnerships and families.[8] These complex disruptions combine various cognitive losses in ways that deeply affect the capacity of the PD couple to sustain a mutually effective relationship as the disease progresses.

---

8 : *https://parkinsonsdisease.net/symptoms/cognitive-changes*

Relational Changes

No marriage is perfect, but many, maybe even most, are "good enough." In a good enough marriage, we rely on our partners to show enough caring about things we value to be responsive to us. Still, eventually changes in the PWP's brain start to make things different in even most well-functioning marriages. These changes seem to be gradual, so it is hard to pinpoint a specific moment when things happen. Yet, over time, things do change. It's not clear how common it is for these relational changes to start before the more visible motor symptoms, but it seems, from what caregivers say, that these emotional/relational disruptions were often noticeable even before the diagnosis of PD.

An early relational change from Parkinson's comes from the impact of living with someone when undiagnosed Parkinson's has begun to change the person's emotional expressions, in face, body, and action. For example, the typical 'still face' of PD, along with increasing apathy, loss of empathy, and less inner control, can combine to make the interactions between a PWP and their spouse a source of sadness and frustration.

Long before the movement symptoms of PD are evident, there can be a real shift in the way a person, who will eventually be diagnosed with PD, seems to react to the normal give-and-take of life with his or her partner. Smiles are not as broad; reactions to a joke or to a loving look start to disappear. The person's inner responses may not change at all, but the ability to show that reaction, to participate in the emotional give-and-take of a friendship or partnership fades. Their partners may start to wonder why things are different. The person with early Parkinson's will feel unseen and misunderstood. On both sides, there can be a general sense that "something is wrong," without either person knowing what is going on or why things have changed.

Later, as PD progresses, some PWPs develop apathy, losing their ability to feel pleasure, gratification, and enjoyment from things that once mattered to them. They cannot feel the satisfaction from the ordinary comforts that were a routine part of life. This effect is dampened for many people with PD since, along with this loss of feeling joy, the PWP may not mind this loss. This seems to be a different experience than someone who has depression, but who may truly notice how joyless life seems and who minds this loss deeply.

One seeming contradiction with the apathy linked to Parkinson's is the intense pleasure-seeking that has been associated with some PD medications. These focused obsessions with shopping or sex, gambling, hobbying or punding (obsessive repairing, assembling, and disassembling things), may be so compelling just because the person's day-to-day life is less familiar and offers fewer interactions or experiences that compete with these intense experiences.

At the same time that the person's ability to care much about the usual satisfactions of life fades, their capacity for empathy also diminishes. Scientists talk about this as a change in theory of mind, a change in the ability to see and understand that other people perceive things differently than we do ourselves. Your theory of mind lets you recognize that other people have wants, needs, and intentions that are different from your own.

A person uses his or her unconscious theory of mind to build up an idea about someone else's state of mind, to read a situation and anticipate the other person's emotions. In daily life we might call this ability empathy. The capacity for empathy makes a person able to figure out how their spouse might feel if a favorite vase was broken, or a parent died, or a long-anticipated movie was coming on the screen. These reactions look and feel like indifference and disrespect and can undermine a partner's confidence in their relationship.

To sustain a positive relationship in a PD marriage, it's the caregiving spouse who adjusts. They adapt their expectations, change their reactions, and find new strategies and different strengths. Still, even the most supportive CP will experience times when things just fall out of balance. No matter how much time has passed since your PWP has been diagnosed, I believe that understanding these relational changes will help you to sustain a healthier connection with your PWP, so that throughout the years, there are satisfactions to be had despite the effects of dopamine loss.

Neuroscientists and neurologists use more technical terms when they are thinking clinically about the non-motor effects of PD. But I want to think about the effect of PD on relationships in a different way, so I use the acronym S.T.E.A.L.S. to describe how PD changes your partner and your relationship. Sleep, Thinking, Elimination, Affection, Learning, and Sex contribute to the ways PD can seem to change your PWP into a different person.

How Parkinson's S.T.E.A.L.S. From Your Marriage

Sleep

If you've raised babies, then you remember the brain fog that comes from ongoing nighttime feedings, and diaper changes. Something similar can happen in life with your PWP. Many caregivers struggle like a new parent because of the restless sleep, vivid nightmares, and nighttime incontinence that are common in PD. Waking up every few hours to help your partner to the bathroom, to calm his nightmares, rub his aching legs and feet, or monitor impulsive nighttime behavior can exhaust a caregiver. You need your sleep. Few of us can feel decent or function effectively without regular uninterrupted sleep. Yet it seems to me that many Caregiving Partners are uncomfortable asking for help with this problem.

These symptoms arise in one of the most private places in our homes, the bedroom. Maybe that is why we think we should manage these nighttime problems on our own. Calling in help, whether from other family members, or from a paid caregiver or service, might feel like an unacceptable violation of our marital privacy. However, remember that the first intruder into your bedroom is Parkinson's itself.

Sleep disruptions are a common symptom of Parkinson's. The brain changes can make a person struggle with falling or staying asleep. Some PWPs sleep during the day, which makes it harder to stay asleep as night, as well. Vivid dreaming, calling out loud, physical activity during sleep, and Restless Leg Syndrome are all linked to Parkinson's. Going to bed with a partner who acts out their dreams and who may even mistake you for the villain in a nightmare can make caregivers approach bedtime with a sense of dread. Adding in the restlessness from nighttime leg movements, inability to turn over or adjust their own bedcovers, and nighttime incontinence can make your nights exhausting. Sometimes adding a bedside commode or urinal, or an external male catheter,[9] can be enough to allow you each to sleep with less disruption. But when the nighttime interruptions persist and rob you of the rest you need to function well, it's time to think about what help you need and where to find it—especially if you also work outside of your home. You and your family need the money you earn, and you may need the personal satisfaction you get from working, as well. And for certain, you need to have slept to function well at your workplace.

So, what are you to do? Some Caregiving Partners decide early on that having separate bedrooms is necessary. This is a painful and difficult decision to have to make, more so because you might need to make it unilaterally, and over your partner's objections. It is unlikely that your PWP is going to welcome having you sleep somewhere else—and when you do make that decision, it can feel like a distinct breach in your relationship, as if you are the one withdrawing.

Here's why I think this is so hard. Over time, you have been slowly experiencing how Parkinson's is making your partner less accessible to you. You've been living with your partner's loss of facial expressions, a lower level of interaction and warmth, less interest in, or ability to do the activities you once enjoyed together. Like many CPs, you have worked at keeping your partner from feeling the impact of these changes. You might have recognized that it would be futile and even heartless to point out to your partner how little he or she has been able to give you. Or you may have been vocal about your need for more participation, more conversation,

---

9 There is also an external female catheter on the market, but it's much more expensive than the male version.

more of their presence in your life. Whether you've been silent or vocal about the changes in your relationship, the decision to move to a separate bedroom is simply one more in a progression of losses of intimacy. For your partner, however, sleeping apart may be the first thing that makes him or her really notice how your relationship is changing. The objections you hear from your partner may be the very ones you have wanted to express for months or even years.

In this, as in other situations, you cannot wait for your PWP to agree with your decision. It is awful, but real, that your best response may be, "I know you don't like this. I don't like it either, But I do need my rest, and to do that, I need to sleep down the hall. It might feel like I don't love you, but I do. I have just decided to sleep in a different bed."

Maybe you will be able to find time to lie down with him at another time during the day, for his comfort and for yours. This may give him a measure of reassurance, but sadly, if his memory is also failing, you could have napped together in the middle of the day, and by bedtime, he will have forgotten it happened at all.

Thinking

It's been going on for a while. Your husband used to be able to do a complicated job, balance the checkbook, operate the TV remote, use power tools to install a shelf, replace a burned-out light bulb, keep his medication in order and remember to take it on schedule, find his way to the mailbox, do a load of laundry (maybe), and make a cup of coffee or a sandwich. Now, bit by bit, he can no longer do these things.

It is still not clear what causes a person's brain to lose the ability to make and to use dopamine and why the extent of the changes is not the same from person to person. Whatever unknown causes have created your partner's Parkinson's, what you notice is how PD changes your partner's thinking and what that means for your life together. Parkinson's doctors will say that PD affects *executive function*, the mental skills needed to carry out plans and goals. They know that it changes memory, insight, judgment, attention, planning, speech, and other cognitive functions. Caregiving partners will just say that their partners can't think the way they used to, the way they should.

If your partner can't tie his shoes because his fingers are stiff, it is fairly simple for you to tie them for him, or to go online and order shoes that slip on or use Velcro. It's another thing altogether if he cannot tie his shoes on his own anymore, but he doesn't know that he can't or thinks he just needs to cut the laces off or to throw away expensive sneakers because "they don't work." It's even harder if he refuses to change to slip-on shoes because he doesn't recognize the difficulty is coming from his PD, or yells at you and call you stupid because you didn't fix his shoes. These sorts of changes in thinking can make life as a caregiving partner exhausting and demoralizing.

It's a rough transition from having a partner who is a functioning adult with physical limitations to having them think more and more like a youngster or small child. It's to be expected that, going through this change, you might feel that you have become responsible for an adult-sized child-like dependent person, which makes you feel sad, abandoned, and even angry.

This kind of caregiving causes you to take on more than the physical functions that your PWP can no longer manage. You also have to take on mental functions he can no longer do. When your partner can't figure out how to make a simple cup of tea or put away the groceries, when you have to remind him to take his pills and not to eat the rind of his orange—this is a different challenge.

Added to these cognitive changes of Parkinson's are the memory losses. As PD robs the person's brain of its ability to function fully, they stop being able to store and to retrieve memories. Not only will the person forget to do the thing that you remind him about—"Don't forget your pills at six, honey"—but also, they can forget events in the recent past. They'll ask, "When are we going to the mailbox?" when you've just come back an hour ago. And as things progress, older memories can get lost as well.

It is hard to be asked, over and over, the same question. However, if your partner cannot hold on to something you have told her—for instance, "We'll have pasta for dinner tonight"—but she is hungry, can smell what's on the stove, and wants to know, you'll be asked over and over, "What's for dinner?" Then again, in a very few minutes, "What's for dinner?"

It's as if the information just moves past her brain, that it just "drives by," but doesn't stop and stay. Each time the thought "What's for dinner?" comes to her, it is a new thought. She can only get the answer by asking. It's not stored in her brain, and she really doesn't know. If this happen to you, try to find your way to being unsurprised and recognize this: she really doesn't know.

I found that once I understood that I was supplying information only for the moment, and not giving my husband information that I expected him to store and recall, it was easier to just state the answer, repeatedly, "Mac and cheese for dinner tonight. It will be ready soon." He could not change the memory loss that had happened to him. Instead, I had to change my idea that telling him something would mean that he could store the information and call it up when he needed it.

Repeating the same answer over and over again is not conversation, and it doesn't give much back to you, but it is what your partner needs. Even if you write your answer on a whiteboard in the kitchen, he may not be able to remember that the answer to the question "What's for dinner?" can be found by looking on the wall.

Making this adjustment, becoming your partner's "external memory," is helpful for him, and also represents another loss for you. Instead of the response you might hope for—"Oh good! I always love it when you make that!"—you get the repeat of the one question over and over again. It's not his fault. He is probably not aware that he asked before, and he won't understand your growing impatience. I think it can help if you can tell yourself the truth about what is happening and thus give yourself permission to become a different kind of partner, too.

When you hear that Parkinson's causes changes in thinking ability, what comes to your mind are probably the changes I've already mentioned— understanding, planning, remembering and problem solving. Yet these changes also apply to thinking about himself, and to awareness of the human world around him. These changes can cause a person with PD to be unable to make a mental map of spaces, relationships, or of other people's wants, needs, and feelings.

You may notice that your PWP moves differently in space. My husband used to stand very, very close to me; it almost seemed he thought that he and I could occupy the same space, the same seat on the couch. If he was having trouble with shaving a spot and asked for my help, he could not understand that he should not turn away from me and look in the mirror but needed to turn his face toward me.

Another way these changes show up is in the loss of *if-then* thinking. Researchers have found that people with PD are less able to consider ideas about things that could happen but have not happened yet. Particularly scary is the situation that occurs when a PWP cannot recognize that the changes from Parkinson's mean that they can no longer drive safely. If your PWP cannot see that continuing to drive is a danger to themselves and to other people, then you may need to recruit the MDS to say that it is time to stop driving, or even to make the decision on your own to "lose" the keys, to disable the car, or to park it away from home and say that it is undergoing repairs.[10]

In this and many other ways, PWPs lose the ability to observe their own behavior and to see how what they do and say affects the world around them. These cognitive changes can look like selfishness and disregard for your feelings. A PWP might get a glass of water without offering to get one for you, too. The person with PD might hear you say, "I love you," and have no idea that you might want to hear "I love you too." PD has robbed him of the ability to turn his mental attention away from himself

---

10 Professional caregivers sometimes call these untruths "therapeutic fibs."

to others. If he is able to get out of the car by himself, he may simply walk away, without noticing your effort to carry the shopping from the car. It feels like rudeness and disrespect, but the idea is simply not there. The PWP can no longer think his way from "he is carrying a lot" to "my hands are empty" to "I can carry something." It's maddening to have to tell a grown person—who at one time may have been attentive and considerate—that your arms are full and you want and need his help. It's maddening but giving him calm information about what you need him to do is more likely to work than just expecting him to recognize what is going on and to then figure out what to do.

In ordinary words, it seems clear to you that your PWP no longer cares about what you feel, what you need, or how his behavior or comments affect you. Still, it is closer to the truth to say that the places in his brain where his mental map of other people's needs should reside are simply gone. The place where "my partner's feelings" would be recognized and understood is just not there. You now have to provide direct information about what you need him to do, without expecting him to figure these things out on his own, and without expecting him to hold on to what you have told him. The adapting comes from your side. You realize that he cannot see *you;* he can't *think+feel* his way into understanding your needs, your situation. You understand that even when you point out that you are exhausted or disappointed, he cannot put aside his own thoughts and feelings, his own needs, to respond to yours.

Often you can prompt your partner, in the moment, to do the things that you want and need him to do: to put a dish in the sink, to get out the dog food, put it in the dog's bowl, to fill the water bowl as well; to say thank you for something you've done. But be aware that your prompts are unlikely to lead him to do these things on his own the next time.

Since this is so, you need to take on the job of knowing what you need and learning how you can take care of yourself. Try to be very aware of yourself and your situation. It is important to pay attention to what feels most pressing to you, to how tired you are and how disappointed you feel.

Your partner will lose the ability to notice these things, so you have to notice them for him (and for yourself, as well) and make sure your needs are met, as much as your situation allows.

Making these adjustments, thinking for your partner, remembering for them, planning for them, all while you get back less and less, will call for readjustments in your partnership. The adjustments you make will depend on your personal style and your emotional and psychological resources. When your partner with Parkinson's stops having the full use of his thinking capacity, it is inevitable that your relationships will change as well.

As this happens, it is important that you don't lose sight of yourself. It is a difficult balancing act, to keep your own needs in mind, and we will look at ways to do that in a later chapter.

Elimination

PD affects a person's motor functions, their movements. This is most evident in changes in their in their walking, posture, hand movements, ability to rise from a chair and to sit safely, and other physical abilities. These mobility changes can make it hard for PWPs to move quickly and safely to get to the toilet in time. However, PD interferes with the brain's communication with internal muscle functions as well, which can lead to the loss of control of bladder and bowel functions.[11]

It's tough dealing with an adult who has trouble keeping clean and dry, and it's hard for you as a caregiver to have to help an adult manage absorbent underwear, keep their bedding dry and clean, to help the person on and off the toilet, and clean their body. When you couple these problems in elimination with the thinking difficulties we've talked about, it becomes a greater challenge.

As a PWP loses the ability to recognize and reflect on their own body and own behavior, they may not be able to acknowledge that they've had a

---

11 https://www.nafc.org/parkinsons-disease

toileting accident. This doesn't always happen, but there are some PWPs who push back against your offer to assist them to the toilet and to let you change soiled clothing or bedding. And it is not uncommon for a PWP to deny the need to wear a pad or absorbent underwear.

Notice that I did not use the word "diapers." That is important. Diapers are for infants and toddlers. Using that word with your adult partner can create an unnecessary blow to their dignity. You can try, from the very first wetting accident, to use the word "absorbent." You can suggest that "we need to find more absorbent underwear." Use that language any time you work with your partner to clean him up. Then when you first add pads to their underwear or swap out your husband's regular briefs or boxers for products like Depends, or other brands, reuse that same term—"absorbent underwear"—to describe them.

Your PWP's lower insight and loss of if-then reasoning can make it much harder to deal with incontinence. They may barely understand the problems that wetting or soiling cause you, and no matter how distressed you feel, showing your distress and expecting him to reason his way from "my partner is upset" to "I will do something different" probably won't work. When it's time to switch your PWP to absorbent underwear or to add extra absorbent pads to the bed, try to remove the emotion from the decision. Treat this change as though it is entirely matter of fact. Doing this may make the transition easier.

Can you do this? Some caregiving partners take this change in stride, while, for others, it draws a sharp line. There are resources to make handling incontinence easier. Using a mask has become routine in the age of COVID-19. Adding a dab of Vicks or a scented oil to reduce the odors, keeping gloves nearby, lining a commode with disposable bags, adding a bidet attachment to the toilet, knowing that foamy shaving cream cleans up urine smells, and other tips are often discussed in the PD online communities. Plus, you'll want to know that various companies such as NorthShore (*northshorecare.com*) and other medical suppliers will even send you samples of pads, underwear, and other items to try as you learn to handle this difficult issue.

Some PWPs will insist that only you can help with this embarrassing need. As the PD caregiver, you have some say in this, too. If you need to have other people be your backup in caring for your PWP, then a loving bit of clear information can be helpful. For example: "I know it's hard, and I know you like it best when I help you in the bathroom, but there may be times I won't be able to do that for you, so I trust (this person/ this agency) to be my helper. I know it's not your first choice, but this is what I need to do."

In this and other situations, you don't always need to wait for your PWP to agree or to give you permission to decide. You can inform them, lovingly and with real regret, that you may be disappointing them, but clearly and calmly state that it's a decision you've needed to make.

In fact, I think we make it easier for a person with PD to go along with a difficult situation if we do not also expect them to have no objections. It's much like something I used to hear from my own mother: "We don't have to like it, but we do have to do it."

Affection

It's common to hear Caregiving Partners say, "He's not the man I married." I think when they say this, they are referring to the interactions between them. The changes in empathy and increased apathy that I mentioned earlier can be such a big change in a marriage that the PWP begins to seem like a stranger. These changes have their impact in a variety of ways.

Dr. Gary Chapman[12] pointed out that not everyone gives and receives love in the same way. These five "love languages" (words of affirmation, gifts, acts of service, quality time, and physical touch) are specific ways

---

12 Chapman, Gary. *The Five Love Languages*. Northfield, 2004.

that we show our love to our partners and how we hope to feel their loving presence in our lives. Parkinson's, with its range of effects on the brain and on behavior, can disrupt these expressions of love. Whatever your "Love Language" is, you may discover that there is less and less of the kind of loving expression that you once counted on to let you feel that your partner loves you.

Words of Affirmation may be your love language. The little note left on your car seat, the comment at the end of a meal you've prepared, a compliment on your outfit, or an acknowledgment when you've helped with one of the physical needs of Parkinson's mean a lot to some of us. These gestures feel most fulfilling when we don't have to ask for them, when they spontaneously come from our partner. On his own, he puts his appreciation into words.

But Parkinson's impacts a person's ability to initiate action—to have an idea or an impulse and to act on it. As initiation fades, you might find there are fewer times when your partner's love is put into words. He may experience your presence and your care as reassuring and supportive, but PD will stop him from letting you know this, and you start to feel unloved.

If your love language is *Giving and Receiving Gifts,* you will notice that your partner may be less able to buy or create things for you. She cannot get to a store independently. She may not be able to remember when your birthday or Valentine's Day is coming; small "just because" gifts stop coming as well. Even harder, when you give your partner gifts, there seems to be little appreciation of them. Your partner's Parkinson's still face doesn't show your partner's pleasure at the things you give, and the loss of language and verbal expression, as well as the loss of memory, can lead you feel that they do not even notice your gifts. In each of these ways you start to feel unloved.

For different reasons, the same thing could be true if *Quality Time* has turned into caregiving time. You may spend all day with your partner, but the way you spend time feels more and more one-sided. Your partner may lose interest in activities or topics you once shared. You do, and do, and do because you must and because you want to, but your many acts of caregiving feel less and less rewarding. The time to just be together diminishes, and you too start to feel unloved.

Acts of Service, those moments when your partner does specific things for you, can also become less common. You might not mind if they cannot do certain chores, or the house is less tidy, or the bed remains unmade. Your partner's loss of strength, of the ability to make plans and follow through, and their loss of skills are pretty clear, and you will get used to taking on physical tasks like yard work, changing light bulbs, making minor repairs, keeping up with laundry, gassing up the car, making meals, or doing all the driving. However, when your partner no longer does some small thing that you once could count on, or no longer shares a treat with you, or eats the last of a meal without asking if you too want seconds, those losses sting.

Physical Touch, the last of Chapman's Five Love Languages, seems to fade as well. Many caregiving partners report that their PWP is less able to convey warmth or affection by physical touch. Sexuality changes, too, and I will say more about that later in this chapter. But, apart from that loss of intimacy, the small contacts disappear: the reassuring hand on the shoulder, the passing touch that can mean a lot. I remember how I ached when my husband stopped making this kind of contact. Until I came to understand that he just no longer had the capacity to do these things, I definitely felt unloved.

Losing these expressions of love may be one of the hardest parts of being a Parkinson's partner. You take on more and more responsibility, you've had to give up hopes and expectations, and to top it off, your PWP has few ways to give back and seems not to even notice how much you are doing.

There is no easy way to keep getting your needs of affection met by your PWP. However, just as you have to take on doing physical tasks for them and thinking for them, you will come to do both sides of the loving, too. It isn't easy. But as you come to understand that your partner can-not remember your birthday, you can remember it for them and recruit someone to help them choose a gift for you. Once I came around to the idea that I had to tell my husband that a birthday was coming up (mine!), I would help him buy a card. It became a different love ritual to go to a store, read the cards together, and have him choose one that was right for him to give me.

After my husband moved to Memory Care, the staff made it an outing to take him shopping (with a credit card I'd provided) to choose flowers and a gift for me and other family members. It was a strange feeling, but for me, it turned out to be easier to help him do the thing I wanted him to do than to just say nothing and feel the absence of any mention of a special day at all. You will find your own way of making sure you help your PWP to give something back to you. You deserve it, and since your partner simply cannot do this for themselves, someone has to help them, even if the someone is you.

Learning

When we talk about learning, we usually think about school, studying, and formal education, or about taking in information or gaining a new skill, and then being able to recall that information and use it in the right moment. Learning is a form of memory—holding on to information and being able to retrieve that information and use it. This kind of memory is often affected by Parkinson's, even when long-term memory remains intact.

Many of us notice memory changes that occur as we get older. It is harder to recall where we've left our keys and glasses, and it's very common to walk into a room having forgotten the reason we've done so. We learn, pay attention, remember, and recall in many ways as we go through day-to-day life: the doctor said to drink more water, and it has been several hours since we have had any; my legs are unsteady so I need to use the walker to go from room to room; milk spoils if we don't keep it cold, so I need to put it in the refrigerator to keep it fresh. Parkinson's can affect any or all of these aspects of learning.

As adults we use our learning capacity constantly when we need to adapt to new circumstances. If the local post office branch has closed, or the supermarket changed its hours, I might not like it, but I will shortly learn that this has happened and will change how I plan to mail a letter or buy my groceries. Similarly, a move to a new house, which requires real adjustment as we learn where things are, is often worthwhile if it improves life overall. Yet, if a PWP's ability to learn has been affected by the brain changes of PD, a change to a familiar routine or to a new location, whether for a brief vacation or to a new home, can be overwhelming. I remember distinctly how disconcerting I found it when we traveled for a family wedding and my husband got lost in the hotel room—he could not find the door.

Another surprising fact about the impact of PD and PD medication on the brain has to do with the ability to learn from mistakes and to learn from successes. We ordinarily expect that a person will tend to learn in two ways: both to do more of things that have good outcomes and to do less of things that result in pain or unpleasantness. It seems that Parkinson's changes this typical pattern of learning.[13] Research suggests that one of these kinds of learning will be stronger in a PWP, depending on the individual pattern of symptoms and whether the person is taking a dopamine-replacing medication.

No wonder caregivers get confused. If your PWP can no longer learn from unpleasant outcomes, then no matter how much you point out that something they want to do has gone badly in the past, they cannot process this information. The bad outcome doesn't stop them from repeating the problem again and again. Even constant reminders of risks (we don't have to call it "nagging") seem to fall on deaf ears, so that we caregivers have to be vigilant to keep our partners safe. Add in the difficulties that PWPs can have with if-then-thinking, and it becomes easier for you to understand why your partner has become unable to keep themself safe.

---

13 Frank, Michael & Seeberger, Lauren & O'Reilly, Randall. (2005). By Carrot or by Stick: Cognitive Reinforcement Learning in Parkinsonism. Science (New York, N.Y.). 306. 1940-3. 10.1126/science.1102941.

Sex and Other Impulses

You've probably heard it said that the most important sex organ is the brain, and yet you may have been taken by surprise by the sexual issues that come with the brain changes of Parkinson's. Many PD couples find easy and natural ways to adapt their sexual relationship as Parkinson's progresses. There are many books, online sources, and audios that help older couples and those with physical limitations to enjoy sex together. (See appendix for some suggested places to turn for this information.)

But not everyone finds it easy to makes these adjustments. You may find that despite having had a stable and satisfying sexual relationship with your partner, things are quite different now. There is no predictable pattern to these sexual issues. Many people with Parkinson's Disease experience changes in their libido, a reaction that some PD medications increase. Some people with PD experience a heightened libido. In some their interest in sexual intimacy or their capacity for arousal may drop almost entirely. Other PWPs may feel sexual urges that are much stronger and more frequent than in the past. In some cases, these changes, combined with the lowering of insight and impulse control, can lead to episodes of inappropriate sexual actions. It's important for caregivers to be aware of this possibility. There have been situations where a PWP will make sexual comments and even advances to caregivers, neighbors, or other people they would normally never have approached.

Many times, a PWP may also approach his or her partner for more sexual activity than usual for their relationship. It can be hard for a caregiver to find the time for or interest in feeling sexual after a long day of taking care of almost everything. Yet your PWP may be reaching out sexually more often. This change is made doubly hard when you are losing sexual interest, or if your partner cannot sustain an erection or achieve orgasm. Many caregiving partners find it difficult to have to help with physical needs, like showering and toileting, and then pivot to being sexual. And of course you do have the right to decide that you do not want to be sexual with your PWP, whether just one specific time, or even for good.

Whatever the mutual give-and-take in a sexual relationship, no one should be pressed to have sex against their will.

There's no easy answer. Some partners have found it easier to help a PWP who feels arousal to address his sexual needs on his own, through private masturbation, or with helping him or her to orgasm, if in fact he or she is able to do so. Others accept that their partner will access pornography, whether online, on video, on in magazines. However, others decide against this solution. It's a very personal and individual decision.

If your PWP does use pornography, it is particularly important to be aware that obsessions with sexual materials and activity, just like excessive spending or gambling, can be destructive to the person and the family. One class of drugs known as dopamine agonists are particularly known for their association with obsessive and impulsive behavior. Two of these dopamine-enhancing medications in particular, Mirapex (pramipexole) and Requip (ropinirole), were found[14] to increase these disconcerting behaviors as much as four times.

As I mentioned above, a PWP's obsessions may extend beyond sexuality and involve excessive spending, gambling, or punding (an obsession with organizing, ordering or fixing things). It is not uncommon to hear about PWPs who have spent their life savings on a stranger they met on a hook-up site, on online gambling, or buying things on TV or online shopping sites or have complicated their home life with hoarding.

Doctors may not be sufficiently alert to the magnitude of these problems and may be unlikely to warn PWPs or their partners about these risks. If your PWP's doctor has prescribed a dopamine agonist, ask him or her to explain the risks and benefits of taking these medications. Also make your own plan now about what you will do to protect your partner, your relationships, and yourself from these effects.

---

14 https://parkinsonsnewstoday.com/2018/06/25/dopamine-agonists-linked-increased-impulse-control-disorders-risk-parkinsons-study/

If possible, try to discuss these risks with your partner before he or she begins to take the medication and together lay out plans for protecting yourselves. At a minimum, create a firewall between your partner's spending and money you and your family need to live. Make sure you have access to your partner's online activity and that a Durable Power of Attorney for financial matters is in place. Get permission to discuss these symptoms with your partner's physician, pharmacist, and other providers. It is surprising to me that drug manufacturers, some of whom have been successfully sued[15] by patients who have experienced the problems, do not make it easier for PD patients and their caregivers to safeguard themselves from these potentially devastating risks.

After all of these ways that Parkinson's Disease takes your partner away from you, what is left? Your way of life will change, but that does not mean you cannot continue to lead a loving and dignified life while caring for your PWP. If you try to hold on to a way of life that will inevitably shift (as life always does) you may find more heartache than if you face these changes and intentionally build a new kind of partnership, a new kind of marriage.

In the following chapters, you will find ways to think about how you want to reshape your partnership, in a way that honors both your needs and your partner's.

---

15 https://www.biospace.com/article/pfizer-agrees-to-pay-off-parkinson-patients-who-developed-gambling-and-sex-addiction-while-on-cabaser-/

Check-in for Chapter Three

Parkinson's seems to look different in every person. In this check-in you will think about the individual ways that PD is taking away from your partner, from you, and from your relationship. Get specific about the things you have noticed about your changing lives and how PD is affecting your relationship. Your answers here will point to intentional steps that you can take to create a new kind of loving and peaceful relationship together.

What is Parkinson's stealing from you, your partner, and your relationship?

Sleep

- How much this is affecting you
- How you have already adapted
- New adaptations you can make
- Help you can seek
- Other thoughts

Thinking

- How much this is affecting you
- How you have already adapted
- New adaptations you can make
- Help you can seek
- Other thoughts

Elimination

- How much this is affecting you
- How you have already adapted
- New adaptations you can make
- Help you can seek
- Other thoughts

Affection

- How much this is affecting you
- How you have already adapted
- New adaptations you can make
- Help you can seek
- Other thoughts

Learning

- How much this is affecting you
- How you have already adapted
- New adaptations you can make
- Help you can seek
- Other thoughts

Sex and Other Impulses

- How much this is affecting you
- How you have already adapted
- New adaptations you can make
- Help you can seek
- Other thoughts

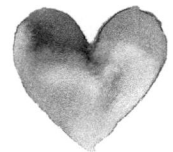

CHAPTER FOUR

Dignity and Love

You are in a PD Partnership, and you probably picked up this book to understand what kind of marriage and what kind of life a caregiving spouse can anticipate after the diagnosis. The difficulties that I described in Chapter Three involve things that may make you feel discouraged, but there are ways to maintain a sense of love (both of loving and being loved) and a shared sense of dignity throughout a long course of Parkinson's. I know because I was in such a marriage.

The time came when my husband was no longer sure of who I was. He asked me if I was his mother. He told me that I was not "the real Terri." When I left him with a trusted caregiver so that I could attend an out-of-town business meeting, he became tearful and told her, "I want the other woman." Throughout all of this—through bowel accidents and episodes of aggression and fear, through falls and his getting lost on the way to our laundry room—I felt his love, and I loved him.

I hope that this does not sound like boasting. Instead, I want to share with you what I discovered, what caregiving taught me about the give-and-take of a committed intimate partnership with a person who needs to take more and more and whose ability to give seems to be fading to zero.

In a healthy partnership or a healthy family, the members each contribute over the years. They put in energy, love, support, kindness, caring, forgiveness, money, work, and countless other things that build up their partner and strengthen their partnership. It's almost as it there is an invisible "relationship bank." From time to time, each partner draws on that storehouse of well-being to get them through times when those assets have become scarce. Some partnerships are rich and well-balanced, with deep reserves in the relationship deposited by each partner so that each can draw on them when the time comes.

Sadly, there are partnership with much less in their "bank." Some are unbalanced, with one partner having made most of the deposits and the other taking more than they put in. Others seem nearly empty with little give-and-take happening.

As you look back on your partnership, how do you feel about this idea? Can you say your invisible bank account is full? How well balanced is it? Has your partner contributed to the internal resources in that bank? How well do you think you have contributed to your shared relationship bank?

I found that when Peter stopped recognizing me, when he lost his sense of empathy, I could look back to how things had been between us when his relationship capacity was intact. Bringing back those feelings, ones based on my memories of having felt supported and understood, gave me extra stamina when he had run out of any ability to pay attention to my physical or emotional needs. Our relationship bank had a healthy balance, which gave me the ability to carry on through the difficult years of caregiving.

Not everyone is so fortunate. If your internal relationship bank is near empty, you will have to find other ways to sustain your love, ones you can rely on over time. It's not common, and it's hard to talk about, but some partners of PWPs do decide, with good reason, that having an outside relationship or even building an exit plan is their best or only recourse.

Love Is a Verb

All around us, television, film, and other media suggest that love is a feeling, something that sweeps us off our feet in an ecstasy of pleasure and connection. However, with maturity and more experience, we discover that love is found as much in the doing as in the feeling.

Sheryl Paul, who coaches people about relationship anxiety, has said, "To commit to your partner is a loving choice, and so you act in loving ways even when you don't always feel loving. Through these loving actions, you expand your heart and grow your capacity to love. This is evidence of love."[16]

If Sheryl Paul is right, then we can continue to love our Partners with PD even when there is little joy to be had in the course of day-to-day life. I believe that even when your partner cannot give back much, you can draw on the long-ago deposits in your relationship bank. Make this a deliberate thing you do to sustain yourself. You might make it a practice to relive one loving memory each day to feel the reality of these past moments of love. Combined with your acts of love, this practice can help you sustain the love in your relationship.

A Dignified Life with Parkinson's

Parkinson's can be an undignified disease as it progresses. Time and again, situations arise that can affect your sense of self-respect and your partner's as well. Still, the planning you do early on can help improve the odds that, whatever the changes this disease will bring about, you and your partner can maintain a loving relationship and keep your dignity intact. This does not mean your marriage or partnership will not change. In fact, you can be sure that it will change. Still, there are things you can do to help maintain your own sense of dignity and your partner's, despite the extreme stresses of Parkinson's Disease. The plan here is to recognize which aspects

---

16 https://www.huffpost.com/entry/love-is-a-verb_1_b_1940731

of dignity are important to you and your PWP to start right away taking the steps that will help you maintain that sense of dignity.

Webster's Dictionary defines dignity as the quality of state of being worthy, honored or esteemed. When you feel a sense of dignity, you feel worthy, and you have the firm belief that other people should respect you and treat you well.

I learned an important lesson about dignity years ago from a coworker when I had just started working with adults who had significant developmental and learning needs. I was sitting at a lunch table with a group of the adult participants, who all spent their days at this program, when Kevin, a man in his forties, let me know that he had a very messy bowel movement in his underwear. I was not sure what to do.

Right away, Javon, a staff person from Kevin's program group, came up to Kevin with a smile, greeted him by name, and mentioned the Yankees, Kevin's favorite team. Javon said he was glad to see Kevin and asked him to come talk about the time he had gone to a game as a little boy. Kevin's face brightened, and he gladly accepted help to stand. Javon, who was clearly an expert caregiver, took Kevin's arm, and they walked away happily, as Javon said, "Let's get you cleaned up, and you can tell me about the time you saw them play."

Even though Kevin was messy, smelly, not in control of his bodily functions, and could not walk without help, Javon kept this man's dignity intact. How did he do that?

The first thing Javon did was to *make a connection*. He greeted Kevin by name, smiled, and invited him into a conversation. *He started an interaction* that was person-to-person, not function-to-function. Javon chose a dignified topic: two adult men talking about sports. Javon never treated the accident as a problem—the solution was what was important. Then Javon *let Kevin know* what his intentions were and *focused on the solution*: "Let's get you cleaned up."

Now, to be sure, Javon was a paid caregiver, and his responsibility to care for the participants in this program ended at the close of each workday—a fact that must have made it easier to show such patience and maturity. Still, his skillful intervention with Kevin demonstrated how these four elements (connection, interaction, providing information, and focusing on the solution) kept an unpleasant situation dignified.

Your Sources of Dignity

Are you currently living a life of dignity? There are so many things in our lives that can challenge our sense of self-respect. Life circumstances, our own illness, poverty, powerlessness, and lack of resources can all make for a less-than-dignified life. However, connection, interaction, access to information, and a focus on solutions, are key to maintaining dignity despite these challenges.

Use these four steps to help you preserve your PWP's dignity now:

1. Let your PWP know you are there, interested and paying attention.

2. Interact on their emotional terms before trying to solve a problem.

3. Give information about how you are going to respond or what you plan to do.

4. Once you've used these steps to set the stage, you can then work toward a solution to the problem you are facing.

You may feel awkward and clumsy at first as you try to use this approach, like trying a recipe for the first time. However, as you get used to connecting, tuning in, and explaining before you act, you can build habits of communication that can make life easier as you develop a new plan for your relationship.

Think about today. Where and when do you feel most dignified, most respected? It might be in your place of worship, or at your job, in your relationship with your siblings or your neighbors, or even in an online community. Even if you discover that you are mostly living without a feeling of dignity, let that discovery alert you to the importance of including your need for respect into your future as a caregiver.

Managing Conflict

As I became a caregiving partner, I realized that I needed to find new ways to handle differences with my PWP. Once he reached a point where he could not easily put his upset feelings of anger or frustration into words, there were times when I needed to take both sides in a disagreement. Doing this, giving voice to his point of view and then to my own, made it easier to use connection, interaction, information, and solution in situations that made my husband feel out of control and afraid.

Kimberly was steaming. Her wife Nan had just presented her with an expensive bracelet for "Sweetest Day," a holiday that Kimberly had not even heard of. It turned out that Nan had responded to a TV segment about this so-called holiday and spent money that was needed to repair the car that took Kimberly to work each day. Kimberly was so mad that she could not even respond to the huge smile on Nan's face. And Kimberly was so upset that she had to say something. This was too big to ignore or to just swallow.

Nan's thinking had become so simple that Kimberly knew her wife would not understand why this gift was a bad idea. For her own sanity, Kimberly needed to find a way to have the conversation, but without devastating her partner. She had to take both sides.

First, taking "Nan's side," she said, "Wow. You really wanted me to like this bracelet—you were trying to make me happy." Nan's smile broadened— giving Kimberly a sight that had been rare since PD took hold. "And you want me to be happy about it."

"Yes. It's pretty! You're pretty," Nan said.

Then, Kimberly spoke for herself. "I want to be happy too. But we need the money to fix the car." Nan's face fell, but Kimberly continued. "You want me to keep the bracelet." Nan brightened. "But I can't."

And with these words, Nan began to sob. "I can't do anything right. You hate me."

And Kimberly feared that out of her own feelings of sadness and loss, Nan would begin to rage. She kept her voice low and reassuring. "No, I don't hate you. I love you. And you gave me this beautiful bracelet because you love me."

Kimberly offered a solution. She put the jewelry on her arm. "Let's take pictures of you, and me, and the bracelet."

And after taking nearly a dozen pictures of the two of them, with the bracelet prominently displayed, Kimberly put the bracelet back in its box and resolved to return it to the store the next day.

"I'm so glad you wanted to give me something beautiful," she said to Nan. "And now we always can see this picture. I'll print it out and put it right over here."

An Honest Assessment of Your Relationship

What about your relationship bank? If you look back to the time before PD entered your life (which could have been long before the actual diagnosis was made), what was the balance of deposits and withdrawals? Whether the bank was full, or nearly depleted, can you think back to loving moments? You may have memories of the give-and-take of a loving marriage. Or you may remember that there were more hopes and wishes than actual loving times. In either case, or in some spot in between these two, you entered into your marriage or partnership for your own particular reasons. Let yourself recall the best elements of your marriage—the actual ones and the ones that were hoped for.

Let yourself fill your loving heart with the best of your relationship and fill yourself with the knowledge of your own capacity for love.

In this chapter I ask you to tell some hard truths. One of the hardest is that some relationships may not have foundations of trust, shared values, or respect needed to ease the way into a PD caregiving relationship.

PD reduces a person's power in many ways. The ability to earn a living or to take care of routine chores at home will start to fade away. The person's body shakes and freezes and is not under their control. Thinking is slowed and confusion increases. The person's mood may become darker and depressed. And if a person, all their life, has expected to be in control—to be the leader in the family, the one in charge—as Parkinson's takes that away, their reactions may be difficult to predict.

Whatever the structure of your marriage, it will change over the course of life with Parkinson's. A highly structured relationship, with sharply defined yours-and-mine roles and responsibilities, will certainly change as PD progresses. If your relationship has been highly structured, controlling, or even overtly abusive, you may have to think now about how you will manage as your partner with Parkinson's loses ground in physical, emotional, economic, and functional ways. You must set the expectation that your partner treat you in the best way they can, not the worst they can get away with.

This is not an easy conversation to have with yourself. Still, thinking right away about what you will need to be able to manage can only set you onto a better path. Whether the adaptations mean having a clear plan for removing access to firearms or power tools as the PWP's judgment diminishes, deciding on home renovations, or moving to a different locale closer to family or heath care, start thinking about that soon.

Along with these things comes planning for skills and knowledge you will need. Perhaps a key thing to consider is that you may never had needed to learn to drive. If you have not wanted, needed, or been permitted to drive, start thinking about how it will be if your PWP can no longer drive. Having a driver's license will be essential for most caregivers, so if you don't have one now, start learning. Many communities have a branch of AAA, the American Automobile Association, which can guide you to driving lessons at a reasonable cost.

Other preparations that you may want to make will come at the advice of your elder law attorney. Start early on to create financial stability and independence for yourself.

If You Are Thinking About Leaving

Sometimes Parkinson's is diagnosed just as you are on the road to leaving an unsatisfactory relationship. You may be waiting until your children finish school, or the house is paid for, or until you are vested in a pension or for some other milestone. You might also just be waiting to see if things in your marriage or partnership will get better. I do not know of any specific research, but I suspect that few relationships improve after a controlling, indifferent, or abusive person is diagnosed with PD.

On the other hand, it may just be that you know that caregiving over an extended period is not sustainable for you. Whatever your reason, you do not have to stay just because your partner has this new diagnosis.

That being said, you may choose to stay because there are costs to leaving: not just financial costs, but emotional costs, community costs, spiritual or cultural expectations that are important to you, or because the alternatives to remaining in the relationship are even worse. Whatever you decide, you are entitled to make decisions that serve you and your values as well as those of the person with Parkinson's.

I firmly believe that maintaining a PD life with dignity and love for your partner can only happen if you are also honoring your own need for dignity and love. And doing this requires looking for the "down and dirty" truth about your partnership. Either in your mind or in a journal, fill your heart and your pages with what you know about the best of this relationship. As you do this, don't ignore the hard times, whether they were moments or months. Acknowledge them, then turn a light onto how even the difficulties reveal the best of your own capacity to love. Think about how you want to honor your commitments, your traditions, your partner, and yourself. Gather what you know about yourself and your partnership at its best to make a platform on which you build your caregiving life.

Taking this mental stance allows you to act from love. I am absolutely not suggesting that you act in martyrdom. Instead, use these questions to discover what you have done and what you can continue to do with an open and loving heart. By doing this exercise, you will have the chance to discover where and how you will need to reach out for help and even to just say "no" to some aspects of this caregiving life.

This process will let you offer all of what you can offer and to honor your own need to say, "No, I don't do that," as well.

Check-in for Chapter Four

No matter whether your relationship bank is full to overflowing, or seems mostly drained and nearly empty, there is love and respect to be found, even if you have to seek them out. It's especially important to remember that these essential elements for emotional well-being are due to each of you, not only to your PWP. Use this check-in to help improve the emotional stores you'll need.

Your Emotional Bank Account

- What is the status of your invisible bank account?
- Can you draw on a strong balance, with mutual deposits of love, energy, and support from each of you?
- To add to your emotional bank, make sure that every day you say something loving to yourself. Start now and write down one loving statement from you, to you. It may seem insignificant to do this—but try it. It probably won't hurt.

Expecting Change and Preparing for It

- Once you expect your relationship to change, you are prepared to respond to these changes in ways that will help maintain your own sense of dignity and your partner's, despite the extreme stresses of Parkinson's Disease.
- Which aspects of dignity are most important to you?
- How will you honor yourself for the ways in which you carry out the hard parts of caregiving?

Write a Mantra for Yourself

- Many people use a repeated word or sentence, sometimes called a mantra, or mental tool, to strengthen their personal resolve, concentrate their minds, and to help reframe difficult situations.
- You can create your own mantra by writing out things about yourself and your life that you value. In the spirit of fake it 'til you make it, your mantra can express something that you want to be true, even if it does not feel true today. Experiment with creating a mantra here.
- If this seems impossible, then start with this mantra, say it aloud, and then fix it up as you go along so that it reflects what you want for yourself: *I am doing a heroic job, under stressful and trying circumstances, and what I am doing matters!*

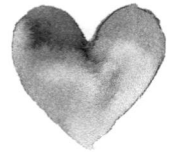

CHAPTER FIVE

Caregiver Capacities or What You Can Do

I ended Chapter Four by reminding you that there will be things that you cannot do. But what can you do? Every person with PD has a unique and changing set of symptoms and capacities. The same thing is true for caregiving. You are one caregiver, a person with your personal style of interaction and your unique set of skills and strengths.

You will find that PD caregiving creates a peculiar kind of intimacy, built from an intense level of involvement and from the way that, over time, we find ourselves losing touch with other people and outside activities that had been a part of everyday life. We each come to this new, demanding role with our personal history of experiences, stresses, accomplishments, and self-expectations. This starting point will include your capacity to adapt to change, your tolerance for isolation, and your own sense of generosity and obligation.

Both Sides Now

Parkinson's robs your partner's brain of the ability to imagine what someone else's mental and emotional state might be. Empathy is not exactly mind-reading, but emotion-reading, meaning-reading, motivation-reading. The gradual loss of dopamine shows up as a slow erosion of these elements of healthy and balanced human relations. Over time, you strain to maintain your relationship, using your emotional resources more and more, while PD blunts your PWP's ability to notice your feelings, or his own.

It's especially hard that, with PD, the person's capacity to participate in the normal give-and-take of a relationship does not just fade away. Instead, it drops out in bits and pieces, skipping a beat here and there, in ways big and small. Many times, and before PD is even diagnosed, a caregiver starts to notice these unexplained changes in her relationship. One day, the PWP is her usual self. A few hours later, for no apparent reason, the PWP may seem to be disengaged and indifferent. Then, maybe after a good night's sleep, or for no reason you can detect, your partner is back to normal. It's not uncommon for these drastic changes to a fracture a relationship, sometimes even leading to a separation or divorce. Unless you were already familiar with PD, you might not have recognized that changes in your partner were early signs of a brain disorder.

Even after the PD is diagnosed, there are more confusing changes. One minute, you feel the presence of a diminished but still recognizable partner. The next, a harsh and critical substitute appears. Then just as you are finding a way, despite this disconnection, to keep the emotional distance you need to go on being helpful and kind to the PWP, it seems he is back and expecting you to be your usual self. Back and forth, caregivers have to reach out, pull back in order to hold on to our self-esteem, and then extend ourselves again. Communicating effectively with a partner who has PD requires a flexible approach as we struggle to adapt in ways to meet our own needs and our partner's as well.

Harvey Karp, a pediatrician who teaches parents how to use empathy to communicate with their toddlers, offers a strategy that helped me stay connected to my husband when his Parkinson's made him seem more like three than eighty-three. The basics of Karp's technique are simple, and they help adults build better communication with a person who wants or needs something but cannot communicate that need effectively. Karp recommends letting the person, whether a child or an adult, know that you understand what they are saying by matching both the meaning and the emotion, the "music," in what they are communicating.

Matching both the music and the meaning can be especially helpful in your interactions with your PWP. He or she may have become less able to recognize or understand his or her own feelings. Putting words to the person's upset while also matching their emotional tone can lead you to talk to each other in calmer and more effective ways.

In practical terms, using Karp's way of connecting with the PWP helps strengthen our own capacity for empathy when the PWP's is fading. We put words to something the person cannot express for himself. Use your ability to think/see/feel your way into the PWP's moment and to reflect back to him, in words and in your emotional tone, the things he cannot say for himself.

Understanding the PWP's expression, his feelings, wants, and needs, is not enough. You also must pay attention to your own thoughts, feelings, wants, and needs. Doing this is important for maintaining your caregiving capacity over the long haul. The less your PWP can pay attention to what you need, the more you must be aware of your own most important needs and wants.

Some caregiving spouses seem to feel that their marital vows mean that they must use of every bit of their own capacity, and only when they are worn thin, when every bit of strength is depleted, do they reach out for help. Sadly, in that moment they may feel that they have been defeated, that Parkinson's has, in some way "won." I see things differently.

I think it is better to learn to pay attention to both sides, your partner's side and your own, as early as you can. Think of it this way: when Parkinson's has dimmed a person's ability to care for his spouse, then you must do this for him. Taking care of you is protecting your relationship.

Doing this, staying aware of conflicting needs—your partner's side and your own—takes real mental flexibility and emotional maturity. Yet, if you can learn to keep aware of your own wants and needs, then you can more easily sort out when and how you want to balance your point of view with your partner's. The goal is to put aside your own perspective while you give voice to your partner's but doing this without losing sight of your own music and meaning.

This idea of holding your partner's side and your own, taking on his job of caring for you, goes right to the heart of success as a caregiving partner. More and more, you will be doing things for your PWP that they can no longer do on their own. Make sure that you're including taking on your partner's job of loving you.

Lou and Cherry's story gives us an example. Cherry is a small and slender woman, and Lou, at six-foot-three, towers over her. She's always enjoyed the feeling of having her tall and robust husband by her side; however, as Lou's PD progressed, Cherry saw him beginning to fall because of rapid drops in his blood pressure, a common aspect of PD. More than once, she has been across the room as Lou walked from his chair toward the dinner table, only to drop like a stone. He was not injured the first few times, but as his stiffness increased, Lou began to hurt himself—a sprained wrist once; another time, a mild concussion.

Cherry realized that she would never be able to help Lou off the floor on her own. Local EMTs were always happy to offer a *lift assist,* and Cherry learned that using that term let the EMTs know that they should prioritize a life-threatening emergency over rushing to help Lou. It also meant that sometimes the couple waited a long while, even an hour or two, for help to arrive to lift Lou into his chair or bed.

Cherry learned to keep a pillow and blankets nearby, ready to make Lou comfortable while they waited, but by the time that she gave up on trying to help raise Lou on her own, she had put such stress on her own shoulder that she developed lasting damage. Despite Cherry's shoulder pain, Lou became quite impatient when his wife did not immediately lift him from the floor to his chair. Cherry was torn. She knew that lying on the floor was uncomfortable for Lou, and she hated to say no to him. More than once she struggled to get Lou up, further injuring her already damaged shoulder. At last, when Cherry's shoulder damage required shoulder surgery and rehabilitation, she knew that Lou could not help to take care of her and could not even keep himself safe.

Having the Conversation

Ideally, Cherry and Lou would have been able to talk together about these competing needs. Lou was falling often, and each time, he hated how it made him feel to lay on the floor, helpless and uncomfortable. Cherry knew that lifting her husband was beyond her capacities—trying to do so just worsened the damage that she had been doing to her shoulder. But Cherry also understood her husband's needs. She hated to have to tell him, over and over, that the paramedics would arrive "soon" to help get him up, when she had no idea how long they would have to wait. She wished that Lou would remember that her shoulder pain was quite intense and that her doctor had insisted that she avoid tugging and lifting. Instead, Lou could no longer recognize Cherry's needs. Parkinson's had stolen his capacity for empathy. He was uncomfortable, and he wanted to get up— now! Lou's falls might not have been a medical emergency, since he did not injure himself, but they were creating a relationship emergency. Each fall chipped away at the emotional health of their relationship.

With luck, you and your partner will be able to talk about the challenges in your relationship. But you may not actually be used to having open conversations about topics as tough as the challenges that come with a diagnosis of Parkinson's. Still, it will be easier to find your way to a mature approach to PD caregiving if you and your PWP can be clear to each other about what each of you hopes for and what each of you expects from yourself and from the other as you learn to be a PD couple.

Unspoken agreements in most marriages or established relationships set up the roles and habits of daily life. Maybe your partner has always been the breadwinner, the payer of bills, the fixer of loose doorknobs and broken appliances, while your job with home, family, and children made you the primary caregiver. Now as PD progresses, your PWP will have to relinquish some of the tasks and responsibilities you both have taken for granted. You might decide to talk with your PWP about the coming changes or, instead, quietly wait to step in as his or her capacities fade.

Despite not having been employed before, you may have to take a job outside of your home. Or, if you have always been employed, you may have to find ways to expand your income or stretch the dollars to go farther. At the same time, your PWP will have an increased need for help and support, whether he or she asks for it directly, or simply takes for granted that you will provide help as their needs expand. As you take on more, your PWP can do less.

For example, Keenan and Jalina have had a relatively traditional relationship throughout the seventeen years since they married right out of high school. Keenan was never much for expressing his feelings in words, and Jalina understood that he showed his love for her in the way he kept her car's gas tank full, her house and yard in good repair, the bank accounts organized, and the bills paid. However, since Keenan began to show more symptoms of PD, Jalina found herself quietly taking on some of these tasks. She now fills her car so that he does not have to stand unsteadily in the gas station. She has urged her older children to join their dad in doing some of the yard work, prompting Keenan to "teach them, so they will know how when they grow up." Without saying so directly, Jalina is preparing her family for the time when Keenan won't be able to carry out his accustomed role.

This kind of subtle planning may work well for a couple that tends to rely on unspoken agreements as their approach to family life. However, for others it may be useful to talk more openly about the fact that a person with Parkinson's anticipates and even expects that his partner will readily be able to meet all of his increasing needs as Parkinson's progresses.

It is traditional to vow "in sickness and in health." But you must decide how you will fulfill your vow. Think now about what you will need in order to fulfill that promise. Start early to talk about what kind of help your PWP hopes to have or will expect to have. You, as the caregiving person in your partnership, should start right away to think about how you will fulfill that commitment.

Setting Boundaries

It is important that you think about the fact that you will undoubtedly not be able to do everything on your own. One part of your planning can include helping your PWP develop the ability to ask for help and to tolerate delay and discomfort. No matter how hard you try, you will not be able to stop PD from having a widespread impact on your partner. He or she will be uncomfortable. He or she will lose physical and emotional abilities, things that matter to them and to you. You cannot make it your job to keep your partner from ever feeling the impact of such a powerful disease. You are not Superwoman. Your strength is limited. There will be times when what you can do will not be enough. There are going to be boundaries. You will find yours, maybe in the way Cherry did, when her body itself gave way, or maybe in a less destructive manner. Your partner will have times of being uncomfortable, upset, afraid, and angry about what is happening to their brain and body. And so will you.

And, if you have not paid attention to your own limits, you may discover what your boundaries should be only when you find yourself lashing out, when you reach your own breaking point. I've known caregivers to express real regret at losing patience, shouting at their partners, or having let out the inevitable upset that comes with hitting an emotional wall. The risk is that snapping back can become a habit. I think that knowing your limits before they are breached, and planning to get the supports you will need, along with giving yourself permission to simply say, "No, I can't," are all important elements of maintaining dignity and love in your relationship with your PWP. Otherwise, you are only asserting your boundaries once they've been crossed and you've reacted, instead of communicating them in advance and drawing lines where needed.

There are two qualifications here. First, if you do find yourself snapping, see if you can look at the situation with compassion and be patient with yourself. This will go a long way toward establishing a different way of responding to whatever may be provoking you. Second, some relationships may have rested on a lack of boundaries. If that's the case for you, recognize that the process of coming to know your limits, planning the supports you need, and learning how to say "no" may take time. Far from being a problem, this is an essential part of the process, both for you and for your PWP.

It is heartbreaking to recognize how PD will distress and diminish your PWP, and many wives and partners urgently try to find a way to completely undo this reality. We jump in, doing as much as possible, because it is just so hard to witness our partner's skills, intelligence, and common sense fade away. It seems natural that we try to take on every possible chore, jumping up to do small things, anticipating our partners' needs, and being at their beck and call. After all, this is what love looks like, right?

Maybe.

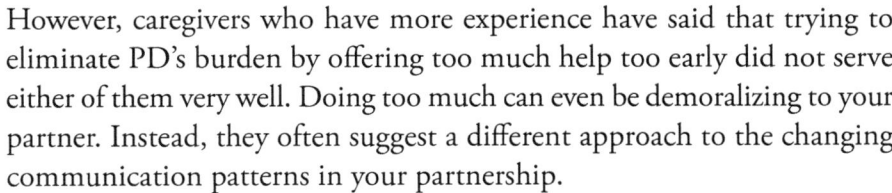

However, caregivers who have more experience have said that trying to eliminate PD's burden by offering too much help too early did not serve either of them very well. Doing too much can even be demoralizing to your partner. Instead, they often suggest a different approach to the changing communication patterns in your partnership.

PD will change your PWP's way of communicating with you. He or she may have developed the kind of mental changes that neuroscientists call anosognosia.[17] These brain experts use this term to describe the way a person loses awareness of their own physical and mental state, their own awareness of the changes that are happening to them. If your PWP has developed anosognosia, she may not be able to recognize that she cannot

---

17 Orfei MD, Assogna F, Pellicano C, Pontieri FE, Caltagirone C, Pierantozzi M, Stefani A, Spalletta G. Anosognosia for cognitive and behavioral symptoms in Parkinson's disease with mild and moderate cognitive impairment: Frequency and neuropsychological/neuropsychiatric correlates. Parkinsonism Relat Disord. 2018 Sep;54:62-67. doi: 10.1016/j.parkreldis.2018.04.015. Epub 2018 Apr 17. PMID: 29709507.

carry out tasks that were once routine. Without insight or "awareness of deficit," your PWP may not ask for or accept your assistance.

One technique that may help you with this change is called "scaffolding," which parents and teachers use to help children who are about to learn a new skill. Scaffolding means that the adult stands by, letting the child do as much of the new skill as possible and only stepping in as a support, a "scaffold" to help with the parts that the learner cannot quite do alone. They watch a toddler's wobbly steps and stand by to offer a hand to hold just before the little one would fall. We caregiving partners can do something similar—we stand by with our PWPs as they do as much of a familiar task as they can, and only step in with a little coaching, or actually take over the task, when the person's skills fail. *Electric trains ??*

Lindell, a very proud and dignified woman, was raised with impeccable manners. She and her husband had always liked to go out for meals—fine dining with friends was an important part of their lives. However, as the Parkinson's progressed, Lindell's ability to manage in the sophisticated restaurants they both enjoyed began to slip. Friends that they went out with often began to notice these changes, and George knew that Lindell was doing things that might embarrass her. He suspected that she was aware of these changes, but that she did not want to acknowledge them. Still, it seemed that they would no longer be able to enjoy meals at the local French restaurants, outings that had been a source of joy for them. So George began to make adjustments when they went out, watching for times when Lindell could not manage something, and, without fanfare, stepping in just in time. Once her ability to decipher a complicated menu faded, he would review the offerings online beforehand and begin to talk about the one or two dishes that he thought Lindell would most be able to manage with her dignity intact. His enthusiasm for those choices would make it easier for her to make that selection in the restaurant. Similarly, he began to sit at a right angle from her rather than across the table. He noticed that she could not always get food onto her fork, and so he would do something that was not typical for them—he'd reach with his own fork onto her plate and in the guise of taking a taste for himself would gently nudge a morsel of the food onto her fork.

These small things may seem like coddling Lindell or denial, but they were a personal adjustment to a very favorite activity for the two of them which made it possible for Lindell to continue to enjoy their regular meals out long after her actual ability had begun to fade.

Doing this can be hard when a person is unaware of the mental changes of PD. It takes a deft approach to offer to help your PWP do a task she's handled easily for many years. You have to find a balance between just taking over and standing by to let the person make a muddle of something important. The way you respond may depend on how important it is for the task to be done just right.

Of course you won't do this all the time. That would be exhausting to you and discouraging to your PWP. There will be plenty of occasions when you will just bring the cup of coffee, help arrange cushions on a chair, find a program on TV, or just pay the bills yourself because you want your PWP to be comfortable and because it may even be easier for you. However, develop the pattern of saying, from time to time, "Yes, I'll help once I finish. Let me know if you get stuck before that," leaving them room to continue to try. This habit will help your PWP experience the fact that even if they have to wait for you to do something they need, they can be sure that you will do it. It will also help them become accustomed to hearing you say, "Not yet."

Over time, it will likely get harder for your partner to wait, harder to tolerate the discomfort of needing something and not getting it right away. Guiding them to tolerate waiting is not being mean. Instead, it is part of building a new kind of partnership in which you take on more and more of a helping role, and they come to accept help in a way that also protects you and your strength for the years to come.

Cherry had to work out her own solution when Lou could not accept that they would have to wait for help to arrive to lift him from the floor. She hated to see how unhappy he was, lying on the floor, so she tried to plan ahead. She loaded movies onto a tablet that they could watch from anywhere in the house, kept a stash of snacks that he liked, and tried to help Lou remain comfortable. But these strategies did not always work, and there were times when she simply sat with him, saying, "I know you don't like it, love, but this is all I can do right now."

What's Your Bottom Line?

Parkinson's erodes a person's dignity and sense of privacy. Stiffness, tremors, loss of balance, loss of control of hands and feet, and overall loss of energy can leave a person with PD needing help with all sorts of personal care. I learned to help my partner shower, to shave him, and once called myself "chief chin-and-bottom-wiper."

You may find yourself taking on similar tasks, since PD affects so many aspects of a person's ability to take care of themselves independently, the things occupational therapists call ADLs—activities of daily living. You will discover where you can help with your partner's ADLs and, importantly, where you just can't. You won't necessarily know where you'll need to step back from helping your partner, and you cannot entirely figure this out ahead of time. Still, it helps to get used to the idea that there will be things you cannot or will not do.

You have to find out what these things are, and start to find resources, as much as possible, to spare yourself from tasks that are just too much for you. You will find yourself doing things that you never thought you would, and you'll also discover things that may have seemed straightforward or simple that now seem impossible.

Some of these decisions will be related to your physical capacities—like Cherry, who could not lift her much-heavier partner from a fall. Others will be related to your personal reactions. For example, as it became necessary, I began to help my husband clean himself up in the bathroom. Of course, that was not a pleasant task, but surprisingly, when the time came, I found it did not bother me as much as I expected. I was able to reduce his discomfort by saying things like, "It's okay. You aren't doing anything I don't do. It comes with having a body."

On the other hand, something that might seem simpler—caring for his feet, trimming nails, and smoothing roughened skin on his toes and heels—was much harder for me. Fortunately, I learned that Medicare would pay for a regular nail trim appointment, so I started using that service as soon as it was clear that he could no longer care for his own feet. For me, cleaning his bottom was less unpleasant. You might not shrink from doing either of these tasks but would hate having to get all wet to help him shower, or shaving him, or some other personal chore. It will be good to discover what you can get used to and what you can't.

ditto

You are entitled to look for help with things you cannot easily do. Even the bathroom clean-up, for example, can be made easier by adding a bidet attachment to your toilet.[18] If, like Cherry, whose story I told earlier, your PWP is taller and heavier than you, it will become more difficult for you to help with his mobility. Many caregivers have caused themselves lasting injury by trying to move a partner who is just too heavy. If the size difference between you and your partner is significant, you can ask his doctor for a referral for occupational therapy to help you learn how to safely move him. There are devices—slide sheets, gait belts, and even Hoyer Lifts—that make this task easier. Your PWP may not report this need to the doctor, but you can send a note without getting permission. Don't wait until you have injured yourself to explore these options.

Whatever limits you discover, start paying attention now to the fact that your PWP is going to need a well-functioning and healthy caregiving partner. As you learn to recognize the things you really can't do (or don't want to do), you will know what resources you need. Taking care of yourself, for you and for him, is an act of love.

---

18 These appliances are not costly and are readily available. Most are not difficult to install. Some even have heated seats and warm-water sprays. You can find them by searching online for "bidet attachment."

Promises

All along, Cherry had vowed to Lou that she would never put him in a home. Now, with her upcoming surgery and recuperation, Lou was going to need care that she could not provide. Still, she and Lou had prepared themselves. Within a year of Lou's diagnosis, they had met with an elder law attorney who had guided them to structure their finances in a way that allowed them to choose care for Lou outside of their home.

Cherry was able to draw on the financial plan that she and Lou had made together as she came to the heart-rending decision that she could not afford to care for Lou at home. Despite shoulder pain that made it hard to drive, she still managed to visit several assisted living and nursing home facilities that she had found, both through local resources and word of mouth from other caregivers.[19] She felt that Lou was too anxious to participate in the early search. Instead, she visited many places on her own, selected the two best options, and only then brought Lou to help her choose among them. Together, they planned the move around the time of her shoulder surgery. Sadly, Cherry's promise to never put Lou "in a home" had made this harder. All along they had considered care outside of their home to be second best, so that it was hard for each of them to think of this move as a desirable choice. Lou felt worried, and Cherry experienced extra guilt over having made a heartfelt promise that she could not keep. Still, paying attention to her own music and meaning as well as Lou's made it possible for Cherry to make the decision that helped them have a better experience overall during this later stage of Lou's PD.

Like Cherry, many PD caregivers are quick to say to their partners, "I will never put you in a home," and to commit to care for the PWP at home for the entire course of their lives. It may surprise you to read this, but I believe that you should never make that promise. You cannot know what may come in the future. Instead, you can sincerely say to your PWP that you will not leave, that you will be by their side whatever happens, and

---

19 For more elder care resources, visit: http://eldercare.acl.gov/

that you will never leave them to live with PD alone. If you can stay healthy, those are promises you can make and keep, but a promise to always keep a person with a chronic illness at home depends too much on the course of the disease and your ability to manage.

Be careful not to use the idea of living elsewhere as a threat—"if you're not careful, you're going to end up in a nursing home" makes these places sound like the next thing to prison. And then if you do have to make this tough decision, you've already made it seem like a terror and a defeat. To be sure, there are awful situations in some caregiving facilities—and it doesn't take much searching online to find videos and news stories about these horrors.

But the truth is that there are many dedicated and compassionate workers who take care of sick and aging people all over the world, not only in in the most expensive private-pay facilities, but in publicly funded or lower-cost board and care homes, memory care facilities, and nursing homes as well. The key to finding such a place for your PWP, I believe, is to start early and search broadly to identify the caregiving resources in your community.

In the US all communities have access to an Area Office on Aging—a non-governmental agency that provides information about the many needs of older members of the community. You'll get a broad view of what is locally available. But also talk privately to your partner's OT and PT—ask which places they would choose for themselves. Try to meet the management of places you are considering. Ask to visit and arrive early for your meeting so you can get a feel for the place and the kind of welcome you receive.

Along with visiting care facilities, listen when people react to learning that your partner has PD. Often, people will have a story to tell, and by giving them time to talk, you are doing your research. What worked for them? Where did someone find good care? Are there places to avoid? Word-of-mouth recommendations are valuable, coming from people who can tell you about their experiences and the experiences of their loved ones. When you have found facilities to consider, remember that many will allow you to make a relatively small deposit to hold a place on their waiting list.

This kind of investigation lets you know what is available in your area. If you are thinking about a move to a new area, find out beforehand what the assisted living and memory care facilities are like. You may never need them, but I wish you the pure blind luck we had.

Almost five years after we had moved a thousand miles away to a new town, a new facility was built—only two miles from our house—a memory care facility that gave Peter excellent care for the last two years of his life. Still, planning is better than luck, and by starting early, you will be able to think about what you might need and to make decisions without the urgency that comes in a crisis. Calm decisions, made before you need them, will help you have the best day-to-day life with PD.

Check-in for Chapter Five

Are you a natural caregiver? Some of us are. And others of us feel that we are pushing against our own inclinations in order to become the caregivers we want to be and that our PWPs deserve. And no one can perform every aspect of caregiving equally well. This check-in has three parts. Together, they will help you identify your sturdiest capacities and the ways in which your caregiving life will be strengthened by seeking other caregiving supports you will need.

Part I—Are you a natural caregiver?

- **Adaptability.** Are you a roll-with-the punches sort of person, or do you know that changes in your routine and habits make you uncomfortable?
- **Tolerance for Isolation.** How important is it for you to have an active social life? Are you an introvert who is perfectly happy at home with a book or video and a favorite beverage? Will you find it hard to spend many days and evenings at home with your partner, without the social outlets you are used to?
- **Generosity.** Some people are givers by nature. Caregiving becomes a natural extension of their usual way of interaction. Others are less patient with setting aside their needs to make someone else comfortable.
- **Obligation.** Are you strongly motivated by a sense of duty or more of a maverick who wants to do her own thing?

Part II—TLC for you

- A caregiver requires TLC, tender loving care.
- How much of the job of loving you has PD taken away from your PWP?
- How are you doing that job for them?
- Do you easily recognize when you are "out of gas" and need to stop and renew yourself? Or do wear yourself thin before your exhaustion makes you rest?

- Where else can you turn to receive the knowledge that you are loved and that your needs are important?

Part III–Managing ADLs

Much of this book focuses on the non-motor aspects of Parkinson's. Still, the Activities of Daily Living are important too. Knowing what help you and your PWP need now and will need later can help you maintain wellbeing for each of you.

	ADLs you and your partner manage on your own	ADLs that you want help with now	ADLs that may require help in the future
Eating			
Bathing or showering			
Grooming			
Walking			
Dressing and undressing			
Transfers			
Toileting			

What steps will you take to find help with these ADLs?

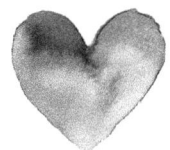

CHAPTER SIX

Planning Your PD Future

Know your Thirsts and Wellsprings

Sometimes people talk about caring for a PWP as a Parkinson's Journey. I'm not sure I agree that it's a journey since we don't really have the destination in mind—and little idea of the landmarks and sights to see along the way. Perhaps it is more like wandering in a forest, leaving somewhere familiar, but not knowing exactly where we will end up. Whether journeying or wandering, we know we will get hungry and thirsty along the way, and that is what you'll find in this chapter: a way to plan for the things you will be thirsty for and the places to refresh yourself. I describe these as thirsts and wellsprings.

All along, we've been talking about the losses that come with PD caregiving. It can empty you, leaving you on your own in a relationship with a partner who may be present in body and in needs, but who has lost a lot of the capacity for relationship. As apathy grows and empathy fades (changes that are all too common in Parkinson's), we caregivers have to look for other experiences to find the things that will sustain us. Caregivers tell us that they thirst for attention, conversation, love, sleep, healthcare, exercise, strength, and information.

These are all important, and having enough of them will make your future and your PWP's future more comfortable, dignified, and satisfying despite the demands of the disease. You won't need every one of these things, but it helps to know which of them will matter most to you. That way you can feel supported and capable so that you and your PWP can sustain this new kind of partnership as the disease progresses.

Start identifying your wellsprings now. These are the resources you can begin putting in place soon. What is important to you? What can you not do without, whether it is a good night's sleep, an hour to read quietly each day, vigorous exercise, time with grandchildren, being outside in nature, or solitude for prayer or contemplation? Something may come to mind immediately. If so, then you know what the things are that you must make room for in your life.

Maybe it has been so long since you paid attention to yourself that you cannot think of anything that would calm or revive you. If that is so, you'll need to explore a little to find out how to refresh yourself. Even if you have no idea of what refreshes you, you probably know what aspects of life today leave you feeling most tired or run down, lonely, or worried. These are your thirsts, and each one that you think of points the way to restoring yourself.

Many PD caregivers make the mistake of thinking that if you do something that you enjoy, if you take pleasure in some activity or experience, you are somehow failing as a caregiver. Too often, we caregivers seem to believe that withholding joy or happiness from ourselves is an act of loyalty to our PWPs. I see that differently. Your distress does not improve your PWP's life. And yet some caregivers feel guilty if they have happy moments or take time to meet their own needs.

For a while I felt this way and thought that even a visit to the library needed to be a hurried trip with no chance to quietly browse the shelves to find a book that felt just right. But one afternoon, I found that I had a little extra time after finishing all the errands on my list. In that brief interval, and with more than a little guilt, I visited a small tapas restaurant close to our house. Sitting at a quiet table with a glass of wine and several small plates of food gave me such a feeling of peace and relief that I vowed to make this little stop a regular part of my occasional afternoons away from the house. This one hour away, with my book and a few small delicious appetizer plates, was a welcome respite and made a real difference in my state of mind and my outlook.

I suggest taking a page from the writer Julia Cameron, whose books, starting with *The Artist's Way*,[20] encourage her readers to make a weekly "date" with themselves, to seek creative renewal. You can make a date with yourself. Every week. Put it in your calendar.

Like Cameron's Artist's Dates, your Date With You is a chance to bring new thoughts into your mind, new experiences to your senses. Even if you are not able (right now) to leave your house to have this date, you can still make this Date With You a chance to break free of the sense of sameness that overcomes many caregivers. One of the positive outcomes of the pandemic-related shutdowns that began in the Spring of 2020 is the explosion of new online resources for a home-bound person. There are podcasts, online concerts, plays, museum tours, ski excursions, scientific discoveries, and thousands of other experiences that you can find at home.

If you can get out of the house for a couple of hours, then your Date With You can start with getting into your car, jumping on a bus, setting your feet on your own patch of ground, and doing something just for you. There are only these few rules for your Date With You:

1. Your Date With You must be *out of your regular routine*. Like any big date, think about something new and special for you.

2. Your Date *cannot be productive*. It is not about doing something or making something for the sake of the outcome. If you decide to bake bread for your Date, make that loaf because of the delight

---

20 Cameron, Julia. *Artist's Way: 25th Anniversary Edition*. Penguin Books, 2016.

you find in the scent of freshly kneaded dough, the sheer pleasure of working flour, yeast, and milk into a silky mound that will fill your kitchen with delectable smells. If other people love your bread, that's an extra benefit, but that is not the reason for your date. Your date is with you and for you.

3. Your date is *not for caregiving.* If you find it impossible to find a reliable person to stay with your PWP so that you can go out of the house, then you might decide on an at-home activity but set your date for "a time when Jay is asleep in the daytime." Then, when the time comes, ignore the dishes in the sink or the dust bunnies in your corners (trust me, they will be there later). Look at your calendar to remind yourself of your activity and get started. To help you with ideas, look at Appendix 3 where I've included a number of ideas for Dates at Home.

Your date is a commitment to yourself. Please take this weekly Date With You as seriously as you would take a therapy appointment, or a visit to the dentist.

Your Dates will become sources of relief, wellsprings that will give you the mental tools to help you maintain your own strength, dignity, and well-being throughout the course of your partner's Parkinson's. They don't have to be expensive. A walk in a park that is outside of your usual area, a visit, all by yourself, to a museum or the local zoo or aquarium, a ticket to the local high-school musical, can be a wonderful date. Most local newspapers report (online or in print) activities available in the community. Keep an eye out for the free days in museums, for art exhibits in your town hall, and for free concerts.

Some of what you experience, and what you learn, will be quite personal. If you can do so in a way that maintains your sense of privacy, write down what you experience. Keeping a personal caregiving journal can help you to build up needed emotional supplies.

Planning how to sustain yourself is part of this process. Start observing yourself in your day-to-day life. Being a caregiving partner is hard, and you are not required to wear yourself to the bone before asking for help. Learn to see when your energy and good nature are wearing thin and find out what you need to do, as well as what help you need to ask for when that starts to happen.

There's a familiar saying that it takes a village to raise a child. It is equally so that it requires a wider community to care for a person with a growing illness like Parkinson's, and this is just as true of the caregiver.

Make Someday Today

Looking back, many caregivers say that they wish they'd done more of the "someday" things earlier. Parkinson's is unpredictable, and no doctor can tell you whether the symptoms will be stronger in two months or in fifteen years.

PD begins to develop for quite a long time before the symptoms take a person to a doctor's office where the diagnosis can be made. By the time you and your PWP know about Parkinson's, the brain changes linked to reduced dopamine have probably been happening for quite a while. Think about the life you and your partner want to have and have it now. Take the vacations, visit the children, move to the one-story house sooner rather than later. Consider this: many of us live our lives holding on for some future: when the children grow up, we'll move to the city. When the house is paid for, we'll retire and travel. Whatever your "someday" might be, Parkinson's can derail these plans, so think now about what you want most to do and do it.

It is vital to pay attention to any plans that assume your PWP's being well and capable. If you live on a farm, or have a big garden where your PWP does a lot of physical work, how will you manage as his strength and balance fade? If you are counting on your partner to help care for a child with special needs, or to manage a business, your plans will need to change.

Build Your Team

Don't isolate yourself. Some couples want to keep the news that one of them has received a diagnosis of PD very private. In Chapter Two we talked about disclosing a PD diagnosis in the workplace. But building your team begins with letting at least a few others know that your partner has PD. As you think about the people in your life and how to disclose the PD, realize that their changes may become noticeable. If you don't help people to understand why your PWP talks less, declines social events, or falls asleep on the couch despite having guests, they may take these changes personally and pull away.

You will be the judge of when you include others in these discussions. Build yourself the care-partner community you will need as Parkinson's progresses. It is common to hear that as a partner's PD symptoms progressed, both the PWP and the caregiver started to lose connection with friends and family members and even with family. I suspect that including your friends in the early stages of managing Parkinson's and helping them understand how they can continue to be in connection with the PWP and yourself may help to keep them in your life.

In addition to communicating with friends and family, storing up good memories can be as important for them as it is for you. I've suggested strategies that you can avail yourself of, like writing notes to yourself or keeping a memory journal. You can also make a private blog to store up reminders of happy moments and experiences. Most of all, take photos and videos—more than you think you'll want—of your PWP just being him or herself, working around the house, getting ready for work, playing with pets, or enjoying a meal or a cup of coffee.

These pictures and videos will help to sustain the two of you and will become precious memories for family, friends, and descendants who have cherished the PWP's love in earlier times. Being able to tell stories and relive good times is as important for you as it is for your PWP.

Check-In for Chapter Six

Have you been keeping a caregiving journal? If not, this is a good time to start one!

Having a private way to take note of your own real reactions, or an online community where you can speak your truth, can help you to step back and sort out what needs in your partnership are going unmet. The caregiving journal is also a good place to work on your personal plan for living a caregiving life.

- In your caregiving journal, record the warmest memories from your life before Parkinson's. Those good recollections can serve you as PD progresses.
- What are your thirsts? What is making you most tired and run-down? What are the deeply felt needs that must be met for you to feel whole?
- What steps have you taken to continue to identify the wellsprings that will supply your thirsts?
- Thinking about your warm memories, you own wellsprings and the ideas in Chapter Six. What might you do for your first Date With You?
- Once you decide on your Date, make a pledge to yourself. Writing down a plan helps solidify your intentions and will help you follow through for yourself and your own well-being and your PWP's as well.

I promise, on behalf of _____ ,

who is my Partner with Parkinson's, and myself, _____ ,

that I will take myself on a date.

I will do this activity : _____

I have set _____ *as the day and time that I will do this.*

(signed)_____

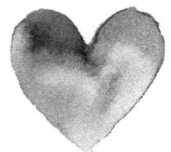

CHAPTER SEVEN

Adjusting Your Relationship

We talked about your internal thirsts and your wellsprings. Now, in this chapter, we can focus on Parkinson's as a couple's disease.

Preparing your relationship is just as important as preparing yourself. The stresses of caring for a partner who has PD call on you to reshape your relationship, together if you can, but on your own if you must, in ways that will make things easier, more satisfying, and as dignified as possible for your PWP and yourself.

To do this, you'll gather, identify, and discover a collection of tools, ideas, information, and habits before you need them. The roles in a marriage vary widely. However, as PD moves along, the PWP eventually lets go of responsibilities or loses the ability to carry them out. Their committed partner will be the primary person to take up these roles. Most PD caregivers will need to take the lead in their relationships. And as PD affects your interactions, you will need to find your new ways of being a partnership. Leadership in a marriage varies. No matter how clear the expectations might be from family, community, therapists or others, each couple finds its own way.

Here are some examples.

Gordon, a person with Parkinson's, and his partner, Laura, have a fairly traditional marriage. "We are the old-fashioned type," Laura says, and both she and Gordon agree that he is the head of the family. Laura asks his opinion, and even his permission, even about things she would very easily decide on her own. For Laura, granting her husband this kind of respect and leadership gives them each a feeling of peace of mind. This style of marriage feels right to her.

Simon and Ezra describe theirs as a mutual partnership. They do not rely on tradition as much as on their individual interests in sorting out who handles various aspects of their household and their marriage. At different times each of them has made more money, and that has not affected how they sorted out childcare responsibilities or household chores. At the same time, they have learned that Simon is better at tracking finances and keeping on top of their bills, while Ezra is a whiz at managing everyone's schedule and making sure the children's homework is done and doctor's appointments are made. In some areas Simon takes the lead—in others Ezra is in charge. The two men like the free sense of give-and-take in their household, and their marriage style works well for them.

Let's look at one more couple, Beryl and Jay. Their marriage is less peaceful and not nearly as calm as the other two. Jay does not like to be crossed, and he lets Beryl know when he is not happy. Beryl has learned to back down to keep the peace, but she is aware that her husband has always kept tighter control of home and family than he might need to. She is careful to let Jay know where she is going and to help him feel certain that she is agreeing with his plans and decisions. While Beryl might have liked a marriage with less tension, she is used to their life together and has learned to manage it.

Each of these couples approach the Parkinson's life with their own style of interacting with each other, and in each of these couples, changes that come from Parkinson's will upset the balance and require resetting the relationship to respond to the PD changes.

The issue of leadership is an important one. As you consider the balance in your own relationship and identify where the sense of leadership falls in your partnership, you will have some new information about preparing yourself as a committed PD partner. As PD progresses, your PD partner is likely to have to step away from many tasks and role that they have routinely carried out.

Of course, you do not want to elbow your PWP out of the way. As much as possible, for as long as possible, you won't jump in to take over things that your PWP can do. Even if their skills have weakened, your PWP can still take responsibility for most of what they've always done. Meanwhile, you can plan to develop the information and skills you will need for when it is time for you to take the lead in your relationship. Just like your elder law attorney will help you prepare for taking on financial and medical responsibilities when that is needed, you can build a plan for taking on other skills and responsibilities.

There is a lot to do to manage a family and a relationship: earning and managing money; household cleaning and maintenance; shopping for and preparing food; managing children's needs and education; care of family, yard, buildings, and animals; managing a family business if there is one; carrying out religious or spiritual obligations; and driving, navigating, and maintaining vehicles. In addition to these responsibilities, when a person has an ongoing medical need, there has to be an organized way of keeping track of medical appointments, medications and prescriptions, going to therapy appointments, and, for times when you will use other caregivers, finding, recruiting, managing, and paying for support from agencies or out-of-home care. All along, you may be cheerleading and coaching your PWP to do exercises or physical therapy as well as managing their emotional states and behavior.

This list is long, and I still may have missed some important tasks that are part of your life. Which of them have been your partner's responsibility? Fortunately, because Parkinson's is varied and progressive, you will have time to recognize where your PWP will start to need help. Among the most basic skills are knowing how to drive and keep your vehicles in good repair and understanding your family's financial position and money management. Starting with these essentials will give you a boost in making sure you can take over important tasks as your PWP needs you to do so.

Other ways you can prepare yourself can include being a bystander when your PWP does important tasks. For example, resetting a circuit breaker is a very small task if you know where the breaker box is and have tried flipping the switches once or twice. You can keep an eye out: if the breaker is interrupted, ask your PWP what they are doing and tell them you want to try.

Can you start your emergency generator if there is a power outage? Do you know how to turn off the water in your house if there is a broken pipe? Who is available to help with repairs in your home? Start now to learn what you will need to know when you are managing most of your household tasks and taking on these added responsibilities.

Losing Your Partnership

I think it is important for a Parkinson's caregiver to start early, soon after learning about the diagnosis, to work out what her caregiving boundaries might be, and for each partner to think about their expectations. It is only natural to want to be there for your partner in any way. It's common for caregivers to feel that they owe it to their partners to give their all, to hold nothing back as their partner's abilities lessen. It feels unloving to take time out for themselves, to continue to enjoy pastimes and experiences that are no longer possible for their husbands.

If you are lucky, you will never experience a partner who no longer recognizes you, who becomes demanding or may even be aggressive toward you. Still, nearly half of people with PD do develop these or similar changes in their way of relating. If that happens, it is extremely hard, after years of being totally self-sacrificing, to set limits. Yet, if you have not built a relationship in which you get to say "no," a relationship where you stop your partner from being unendingly demanding or disrespectful, it will be a much harder challenge to establish these limits and boundaries later, when his ability to cooperate with you will have become much more limited.

Setting limits does not mean being harsh or ungiving. When PD takes away your partner's ability to fully make choices about how he treats you, how he behaves with you, you must carry out those functions for him—doing for him what he can no longer do on his own.

I will never forget the day when, after many times of wishing Peter would reach out to hold my hand, or touch me, or smile at me, I said to myself, "He has nothing for you." This was especially hard because he had been such a connected and considerate husband in the first years of our marriage. However, the combination of his losing the capacity for empathy, the still face that had stolen the simple loving looks I'd come to expect, the loss of the power to initiate action, and the increasing need for my attention and support left me aching.

It had taken a long time for me to realize that he no longer had the brain capacity to show love or to act lovingly on his own. So, just as I had to help him maintain his balance and walk safely when he could not on his own, or had to help adjust his diet, and manage his constipation and balance our checkbook, I also had to help him be a loving husband. He couldn't do it, so I had to do it for him.

None of the websites or books on Parkinson's told me to expect the loss of partnership. They rarely describe the emotional one-sidedness of a Parkinson's marriage, which leaves many PD caregivers thinking that their partners have stopped loving them. Despite how common this experience is, PD caregivers often feel they are not entitled to notice how empty, lonely, or burdened they feel. "Somehow," they reason, "if I were a really good spouse, a good person, I would not mind giving everything I have."

This kind of thinking can lead caregivers to set no limits, to never engage outside helpers, and to make the "no nursing home" promise. Doing this kind of thing means the caregiver is not taking care of their partner's most important resources for the course of life with PD, a capable and active caregiver.

Parkinson's disease, as I said at the beginning of this book, is much more than disease of the muscles and movement. Even in its early stages, it disrupts the person's relational capacity. Part of your caregiving agreement with your husband should address how he can join you in preserving your ability to take care of him.

How to Work with Difficult Behaviors

To set limits and boundaries in your caregiving relationship, you'll need to know what you want. Then you have to know that you are entitled to feel safe, to be renewed from time to time, and to have access to the information and resources you both need to establish and maintain a successful caregiving relationship.

I remember an old song I first heard at a folk concert in the 1960s. It became an anthem of women's boundless capacity. "I can starch and iron two dozen shirts and hang 'em on the line…feed the baby, grease the car, and powder my face at the same time."

Many women, especially, pride themselves—and more expect themselves—to handle every chore and responsibility thrown at them, rarely complaining. A caregiving wife would add to the song being able to manage the family finances, clean up after her husband uses the bathroom and misses, pick him up when he falls, sort and manage half a dozen medications, and more.

However, being a martyr to Parkinson's Disease, without knowing there are limits, and without knowing how to set them, is a way to send yourself down a road to resentment, exhaustion, illness, and deep loneliness. I don't think it has to be this way.

You have probably said from time to time that you love your partner, you'll "be with them," and maybe that they don't need to worry. Still, if you are more specific, your partner will probably worry less. Being specific will also help you.

Becoming a caregiver to someone who is likely to lose the capacity to be considerate, to respect your needs, or to recognize and modulate his own feelings is rarely talked about. I have heard from many caregiving partners that their PWPs become disrespectful, combative, aggressive and act in other problematic ways. Many of us have tried to be understanding and compassionate and to not push back, but I think it could help if a caregiving partner begins, right away, to set the expectations for how their PWP will treat them.

Your PWP may not be agitated or aggressive. Still, sometimes, as the loss of inner control and the failures of empathy and the apathy progress, a PWP's behavior may become difficult to manage. If this happens, many caregiving spouses are taken aback. We try to see our PWPs as "still themselves," so when a new, harsh way of treating you shows up, it is normal to take it at face value—which is a very painful situation.

Alexithymia is a clinical term for the difficulty PWPs have in understanding or recognizing, naming, and understanding their own emotions or thoughts. Not every PWP is going to develop this recognizable symptom of PD. If they do, it causes enormous strain on the caregivers who carry the physical and economic burdens of caregiving as well. Since your PWP may not be able to tell the difference between being scared, worried, lonely, or angry, it can be harder for her to know what she wants and needs and hard to let you know how to help her. Your way of communicating will have to change in response. You can start to build new habits of communication that will help PWP recognize and value when you say "yes" and to tolerate when you say "no."

Since they lose both their ability to read their own feelings and to read yours, you cannot expect that your PWP will know when his behavior is affecting how you feel or what you need. Even telling them that something upsets or worries you may not be enough to improve how they treat you.

As your PWP loses the ability to read his own feelings and thoughts, and yours, there does not seem to be any way to restore that capacity. What you do, however, can affect what your PWP does. And that starts with not simply letting disrespectful or harmful behavior pass because "it's the disease."

I believe that you can alter this situation. You do not have to simply absorb language and behavior that distresses you. Instead, start right away to see these symptoms for what they are, signs of a disrupted brain, and to protect yourself and your relationship from their harmful effects. While you cannot restore your partner's brain, you can avoid the damage that these symptoms can cause to your caregiving relationship and to you.

You'll need two kinds of resources. First, learn the skills that help you redirect and deflect the difficult behavior that comes from your partner's changing brain. Teepa Snow[21] is an online expert whose videos and podcasts will guide you finding more effective ways to approach your changing partner with compassion and sensitivity. Second, you'll want to find a loving way to stand in a neutral middle, keeping your own feelings, needs, and worries on one side and your partner's reactions and behavior on the other. Then, standing in that "middle place," you have to know what you need, what is most important for your own well-being as you guide your PWP's behavior.

If your PWP is losing the ability to read and understand his own feelings, if he cannot tell the difference between his fear, worry, loneliness, anger, or other uncomfortable feelings, they all may be expressed through agitation, angry words, and aggression. When your partner's behavior toward you has changed this drastically, you must make up your mind to respond more to their behavior than to how their feelings about you appear to have changed.

Yes, what you are hearing can be devastating. Still, try to recognize that this new behavior reflects how profoundly PD has robbed your partner of their own sense of who they are and their sense of who you are. In response, recognize that you are dealing with symptoms and not with the person who is your partner.

---

21 https://teepasnow.com/resources/for-families-and-friends/

It is in moments like this that you may realize that it's time to take steps to protect yourself and your partner from the harm that these symptoms can cause. I mentioned earlier that if there are firearms and ammunition in the house, you'll need to consider disabling or removing them.[22] It's also vital to keep vehicle keys, power tools, and other dangers out of your partner's reach. It's tempting to keep hoping that your PWP will come to agree with the need to set aside these dangers. But it is likely that you will have to take these steps whether he agrees with this decision or not. Your PWP may be furious at this evidence of his lost abilities, and you may become the target for rage that properly should be directed to the unfairness of the disease itself. The anger may come your way, but try hard not to let this behavior reach your heart.

Instead, you now will need to give yourself the respect and protection that your PWP can no longer give you. Don't wait until this kind of experience is a common part of your daily life. Instead, when your partner's way of talking to you or acting toward you has become combative or hostile, start right away to set limits and redirect them. Try to keep a moderate tone of voice. Your PWP probably cannot, in a moment of agitation and distress, recognize how what he or she is doing is upsetting or hurtful to you. And what you say will probably not redirect his or her thoughts or attitude.

Caregivers may respond to their partner's shocking behavior with an equally raised energy and sharp voice. They react to unfair allegations of neglect or of cheating as though they were real. At times, his shouted threats, born of fear and frustration, may make you fear that he will hit you.

If you had not known that such distorted thinking is common in Parkinson's, it makes sense that you would argue against it. You are nearby day and night, managing the household, taking care of him. It is impossible for you do to everything he wants all the time. And as for cheating, where would you find the time or the energy for that?

---

22 https://khn.org/news/dementia-and-gun-safety-when-should-aging-americans-retire-their-weapons/
https://khn.org/news/worried-about-grandpas-guns-heres-what-you-can-do/

However, if you have learned ahead of time that these accusations are familiar, and that PWPs often become angry and accusatory without justification, then you can respond differently. You can redirect their behavior and step away from a situation that might otherwise become conflictual.

First, step back from the situation in a neutral way and name the behavior. For example, "You can't find your slippers, and you want them now." Or "It seems like I'm having an affair with Joe." Then take the hard step of restating his feelings or fear to him.

"That must make you really upset with me." Or "Wow! You'd be so unhappy if I did that."

Then you can start to set the limit. "When you are yelling like that, it makes me scared, and I can't listen to you." You can reassure your PWP that you would never hide his things, or be unfaithful, while keeping your tone calm. You are not trying to persuade your partner to agree with what you have said. Don't expect his feelings or reactions to change. Instead, you are redirecting his attention and energy without joining in or amplifying the heat of his worries.

As you redirect your partner's confused thoughts, you can then reset the situation and redirect their attention. Suggest an alternate activity—a snack, a walk, or a new conversation—to turn away from the agitation of the moment. Doing so is a challenge for you since you may still carry your partner's hurtful claims in your heart.

When you reset and redirect your partner's behavior, you are both showing him how to react and building your own new habits of responding. You strengthen yourself and you to preserve your connection with this new person that your PWP has become.

You may feel that giving your partner direction and instruction is disrespectful to them and even that you are treating them like a child. To that I say yes. Like a young human being who has not yet developed empathy, impulse control, or self-awareness, your PWP is an older human being who is losing these essential skills.

Most important, when you are taking this middle ground, you cannot inject your own emotions. This is not an argument, and you are not likely to succeed if you are yelling, crying, trying to persuade, or hoping to restore the pleasant, loving attitude your PWP may have had in the past. Instead, all you are doing is supporting your PWP to follow your direction, direction that you have made simple and easy to understand. Instead of being caught in an argument, you have the chance to succeed in changing this pattern in your caregiving life.

Making this shift in your relationship with your PWP is a hard thing for PD caregivers. You have to find a way to stay calm and dispassionate, to look at the interaction and behavior without trying to change the PWP's feelings. All you are doing is making your help contingent on the behavior that keeps you both safe.

Something like this happened in my caregiving life. My husband was a supportive and loving man, but as his PD dementia increased, there were frightening situations I had to learn to manage. Sometimes, he would get scared and upset as his ability to understand things got worse.

There was a day when Peter became more and more agitated with me. I no longer remember what the issue was, but I know he was falling apart, cognitively and emotionally. At last, he raised his hand as if to strike me. Drawing on my experience in working with adults with cognitive disabilities, I reacted by grasping his wrist and saying, calmly but firmly, "Peter! Don't hit me." I was not asking. I was instructing.

I looked directly at him. "Are you a man who hits his wife?"

He said he was not.

I said to him, "Then don't."

It wasn't easy to take on such a directive and dispassionate tone, but it helped. And the few other times when he raised his hand, I was able to use the same language: "Are you a man who hits his wife?"

Another time, I had to tell him I was walking away because I could not help him if I was afraid of him. I said, "I'm going downstairs for a couple of minutes. I'll come back and see if you are ready to tell me what you need." Then I did just that. I said, "I can't stay in the room with you if I am afraid of you. I'll be back, and we can try again." I gave him just a few minutes and then came to him with bright, cheery voice to say, "What do you need, love?" My positive energy was able to pierce through his distress and connect with him. Clearly, he wanted to be connected with me and wanted my help. By doing this, drawing on my past work experience and long-dormant acting skills, and putting aside my own worry, I was able to reset his state of mind and restore our connection.

Of course, each caregiver and PWP have their own history together, and you will use words and suggestions that remake a connection with your partner. And, depending on your partner's current capacity, you may be able to talk more directly with your partner about the changes that are necessary in your relationship.

Bethany, a caregiver in an online group, told the story of her husband developing a pattern of insulting and cursing her, rejecting her help, and ignoring how hard she was working to take care of him. I suggested to her that she recognize the signs of these relational disruptions of Parkinson's and change the script:

"I take care of you because I love you, but if you wear out my love with hateful words and insults, I won't have what I need to take care of you. It is not allowed for you to be mean and insulting to me."

I told Bethany: "Don't cry, don't raise your voice, and don't ask him to agree with what you are saying. Inform him, calmly and lovingly, that these are the facts and then leave the room. Don't wait for him to agree.

This is *your* decision to no longer accept his hateful speech." Since her PWP could not call on his own innate empathy, which the disease had stolen from him, Bethany had to decide what the limits and structure of the relationship would be.

Once you have decided on a boundary, you must give your PWP simple information about limits. Remember, he is losing his ability to meet your needs, so you have to be the one to do it. I passionately believe it is a mistake for a caregiver to simply permit this symptom of PD to shape the interaction between you.

Just like you help him with other things he cannot do, you must help him respect you and treat you reasonably. Don't wait for him to want you to do this for him. He can't. Instead, decide on the things you expect (within the boundaries what he *can* do) and let him know that he must. He cannot simply have everything you can give without having to experience reasonable boundaries and limits.

Consider this: there are some limits you would easily set. If your PWP asked you to lift up the refrigerator, you wouldn't try to do it. Because you know that is a real limit, you would not struggle internally to try to carry out this impossible task. You would reject his request.

You can set other limits with the same internal certainty. You know what you cannot do or will not do for your PWP. You can say kindly, and with genuine regret, "I know you wish I could. I wish I could always do what you want, but I can't do this. So how else can I help?"

Being kind and clear in this way helps both of you. It gives your PWP clear information about the world around him, and especially about you, his main caregiver. This will help him to manage the difficult process that ultimately he has to go through on his own. No one can bear the Parkinson's burden for him; however, knowing what help is there, without having to wonder, without having to figure things out, will be more reassuring for him.

If you have not known how to set limits with your PWP, and there has been a pattern of this kind of unacceptable behavior, I think you can tell your PWP what I advised Bethany to say earlier. *I take care of you because I love you.* Remember that this is *your* decision to no longer accept his hateful speech.

If your husband has been treating you in ways that harm you physically or emotionally, then a reset is definitely in order. First, you must recognize that your safety matters. I know there are times when a caregiver says, "It's not him; it's the Parkinson's." Recognizing that truth can help a caregiver understand that the aggressive behavior is not personal. At the same time, knowing that it's "not him" can allow you to be clear that you do not have to endure fear and violence at the hands of a person whose words and actions are being directed by a disease process and not by their own will or intention. Certainly, you are entitled to get as much information as you can about steps to take to improve the safety of your home, and to take those steps. Even if you do not have medical power of attorney or a medical release, you can still privately inform your PWP's doctors about what is going on. You may even decide that it's wise to inform local law enforcement that you are living with a person who has a brain disease and that you may need their help to manage difficult situations. You can make a safety plan for you and your PWP. You can tell yourself the truth, so as to not minimize how much fear and injury can occur at the hands of a PWP who is not in control of his own behavior.

It is important to know that this reset involves changing how you understand your marriage. When you know that, despite the stresses and risks, you are staying in your relationship, you help yourself by knowing *why* you are staying. This starts with understanding that if you cannot expect to have your emotional needs met and your safety valued, you can still have good reasons to stay. Then honor yourself for doing this.

If your partner's well has run dry, you will have to find your wellsprings elsewhere (in your loving past, your spiritual life, reading, TV, playing music, taking walks, or friendships). Many of us draw on the emotional bank that was filled long ago to sustain us down the years of caregiving. However, stop looking for warmth and joy, caring, or recognition from your husband if Parkinson's has stolen his capacity to give them to you.

I know this reality will take a while to settle in. You'll cry bitter tears and imagine running away or committing mayhem and pray for a rescue. Get these feelings out. Again, journal—whether on paper on in a computer or the notes on your phone. Tell yourself the truth and love yourself through this process.

Lots of caregivers get help from a spiritual advisor, coach, or therapist to learn about this part of their caregiving lives. Once you are firmly on this path toward acceptance of your partner's relationship disability, it will be time to start gaining a new caregiving partnership with them.

In this new partnership, you won't need to react with as much emotional force to the problematic interactions. Oh, you will still be impatient and frustrated plenty of times, and you may even speak harshly or raise your voice. However, accepting that Parkinson's often causes disrupted relational capacity sets you on the path to managing how your partner treats you without this kind of reaction.

Guiding your PWP to Treat You Well

The time may come when your partner will need even more direction in how to treat you. He won't be able to smile at you anymore; that's gone. Yet, if a greeting in the morning is important to you, then you'll let him know, lovingly and calmly, that it helps you to take care of him if he says good morning. And if he does not remember from one day to the next, you help him. "Good morning, Doug," you'll say, and then, with a light touch, "Your turn now—tell me good morning!" And if PD dementia has progressed, and your partner is not aware enough to respond to these conversations, you'll find other techniques to be helpful. The overall approach to this kind of situation is to remain unsurprised at the changes in your partner and, as much as you can, construct situations that feel better to you and that enable you to continue the hard work of caregiving.

I've mentioned the work of Teepa Snow before. She offers a set of key phrases for communicating with an angry or agitated person with a brain disease. I think these phrases can help you reach in, past the confusion and fear that people with dementia often experience, to make contact with your PWP.

Two of her phrases are:

"I'm sorry. I was trying to help."

"I'm sorry. I made you angry."

Using phrases like these helps you to apply the Harvey Karp technique, mentioned in Chapter Five, to communicate with your partner. They let you reflect to your partner that you have gotten the message about his feelings, about his reactions, and that you want to help. And that is, after all, the main message to give to our Partners with Parkinson's: that we want to help.

Check-in for Chapter Seven

The shifting balance of energy, leadership, responsibility will happen. Instead of always needing to catch up as these changes occur, you can pay attention now to what you are discovering about the changing patterns in your relationship.

- Take a moment to think about the balance of energy in your relationship. How might your PWP feel as his or her capacities start to falter?
- Many couples experience shifts in the balance of their relationship before the PD diagnosis occurs. Are there ways that this has happened to you? Does your new understanding of your partner's emotional changes make a difference in how you feel or clarify why things have changed?
- Have you taken on new roles or learned new skills to help keep life afloat in your household?
- What have you needed to let go of as PD progressed? How do you feel about that?
- How are you creating mementos of your own life? Are you taking photos, making videos, saving small souvenirs of your life? And if your answer is "I'm not," how will you change that?
- If you been expecting yourself to have no struggles and no sense of loss, what can you do about that? What is stopping you from offering this kind of empathy to yourself?
- Which ideas from Chapter Seven will help you take better care of your partner's caregiver—that is, to take good care of yourself?

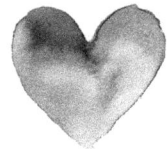

CHAPTER EIGHT

Endings and Beginnings

I hope this book, with its tough truths, has been able to make the PD path more predictable and that it serves to sustain and comfort you and your PWP.

Parkinson's of course, only lets you travel in one direction, and there seem to be only two ways your time as a PD caregiver ends. In some situations, ending the relationship may be what you do. That is a tough decision you may have made, and it shows courage. I'm sure people will be quick to judge. However, your partner's diagnosis may have turned a bright light onto things that have been wrong for years in your partnership. Or maybe you recently met this PWP and didn't learn right away that he had PD or did not understand how much would be required to stay the course.

If this is your decision, and you have decided to end your relationship with the PWP, you are probably alternating between a sense of guilt and tremendous relief at the prospect of having the weight of PD lifted from your shoulders. Still, you have something to grieve too. If you have read this far and made the decision that you cannot do this, I suspect your decision was not cavalier or callous. Not everyone is called to do this; not every partnership affords the conditions for a healthy Parkinson's relationship. Unless you are constrained by religious requirements or cultural limits, no one should (in my opinion) be asked to shoulder such an enormous burden without their consent.

The other way your job as a PD caregiver ends is, of course, the end of the PWP's life. It's a truism that gets widely repeated (and widely criticized as well) that a person doesn't die "from Parkinson's" but "with Parkinson's." I won't get into the technical weeds of this difference. In any case Parkinson's doesn't go away. Dopamine-producing areas of the brain don't get restarted into action, so the course of PD—gradual in some cases, heartbreakingly intense in others—accompanies the person through the end of life.

I have an app on my phone called *We Croak*.[23] Its one purpose is to give its users reminders, several times a day, with different quotes from all over the spiritual and literary world, that we will someday die. *We Croak* is inspired by a Bhutanese saying that remembering, five times daily, that "we all die" brings happiness. True or not, I have been finding that letting my mind rest on that fact has not depressed me. That we all die is something we learn at a young age, and while we are particularly good at not noticing this fact, my experience tells me it helps to let that truth in. That truth is only surprising or shocking if we are holding on to the fantasy that we will live in this life forever. But life ends.

Some PWPs discover a new energy for exercise and motivation despite the distresses of Parkinson's. Others seem to settle back into the reality of the diagnosis. It may seem to some of us that the second choice means losing the will to live. But will is not what keeps us alive. Life has its own trajectory. As it fades, having a false insistence on being more alive than our bodies will let us be is, I think, just a recipe for pain and an ultimate sense of failure. Let your PWP be at the stage he is in and care for yourself as well. This is your partner's process and their stage of life. It's hard, but it is natural and real.

Despite the promises of hopeful researchers and the deceptions of char- latans, there is currently no cure for Parkinson's. There doesn't seem to be much value in spending the healthy aspects of the time remaining in a PWP's life searching for a monumental cure that does not exist. People

---

23 https://www.wecroak.com

have needlessly lost time, money, and health chasing false cures. In my life with my PWP, I found that living in the present and putting our resources into sustaining what was working was the better use of what we had. You can help your partner have a life that sustains and comforts you both, in equal measure, for as long as possible.

Death is a natural and inevitable thing, as Shakespeare put it, an unknown land "from which no traveler returns." Do you know what you think about that? You may believe in some way that you end when you take your last breath, or you may have faith in an eternal hereafter. Whatever your beliefs, finding your own way to treat death as life's inevitable last act may well remove some of the dread.

My experience was that, as his life waned, keeping my PWP free of fear and free of pain was my job. My husband's Parkinson's left him, in his last years, unsteady, frail, and confused. After he recovered from a broken hip that came from a fall, we did spend some time in the search to restore things to the way that they had been, just a few months earlier.

One day, after a strenuous visit to an orthopedic surgeon who was planning to do a hip replacement (which I wished had been done at the time of the fall), Peter became extremely agitated and loud. As we sat in the building's lobby, waiting for the wheelchair transit to meet us, he kept shouting that he didn't like or trust me, that he wanted to die, that he wanted to get away. It was tough, embarrassing, and more than a little frightening.

Trying hard to listen and to understand what he was asking for, I could tell how scared he was. Once I recognized his fear, I used the Harvey Karp technique, adjusting my language and emotion to mirror his emotions. That way, I could join with him, find a way to address his feelings and confusions, and let him know that I understood the goal he could not state for himself.

I told him I knew he was afraid, and that I would do everything I could to keep him free of fear and free of pain. When I made that promise to him in the doctor's waiting room, he became much calmer and said twice, "That's what I want." I think he felt understood, and I felt able to focus on those two goals. Throughout the process of his dying, when he seemed afraid, I reminded Peter that I was there, that I loved him, and that I would help him. That he died peacefully with the help of hospice, pain-free, breathing slowly in my arms, was the most natural ending of our too-short loving life together.

As you think about the reality that a PD life ends, do not be slow about reaching out for the support that palliative care and hospice organizations offer. Too many people make the mistake of thinking that this kind of care is only offered in the last weeks of life. Instead, once medical interventions are clearly not going to change the course of an illness, it is appropriate to get the help of hospice and palliative care organizations to make your PWP's remaining life, even if it is counted in months and not days, as comfortable and dignified as possible. Be sure to search out the local choices in palliative care and hospice organizations available to you, both for-profit and non-profit, so that you can make a choice before this is an urgent need.

The idea of anticipatory grief rings true for many PD Caregivers. Long before the PWP leaves this life, your relationship has shifted and slumped, like a fallen cake, so that much of what was once there slipped away. It is hard to mourn, to grieve the loss of a companion, golf partner, fellow parent, while you are still doing the most personal and intimate kind of caregiving. You've been mourning for years, and yet now you are free to mourn both the person whose life has ended and the person, the relationship, marriage, or partnership that was ended some time before by the effects of PD.

As for what comes next, in some ways, the same factors that influenced your caregiving experience will affect how your life proceeds after your partner's death. You may have other family or caregiving responsibilities that will shape your life. You may still be living with strained finances, or you may be relieved to be able to turn your resources to tending your own health and well-being.

I am writing these words only a year after my own PWP's death. Yet, because I've been fortunate—because he prepared for me and cared well for me when he could—I have been able to turn my attention to my own questions about living the remainder of my life. I hope that what I have written here will help to equip you for this hard thing you have to face. I hope you can breathe, trust yourself, revisit the sections of this book that helped you know yourself better, and reach out into the world, knowing you will do your best—you will have done what you could.

Check-in for Chapter Eight

Neither you nor your PWP has chosen this path, and the overall truth of your individual PD caregiving story only emerges over time. Throughout this book I have wanted to help you recognize the choices that are in front of you, so that in choosing you escape feeling overwhelmed and diminished by the experience of caregiving. That way you will shape the way you carry out the role of caregiver, so that you approach this life with an open heart.

- What are the choices you have made that allow you to continue to shoulder the responsibility of PD caregiving?
- Can you tell yourself why you are taking care of your Partner with Parkinson's?
- If you have decided to leave the relationship, can you give yourself permission to make good enough arrangements for your partner as you reset your own path? What are those arrangements?
- If you walk alongside your partner until his or her end, what end-of-life experts will you turn to for their expertise and companionship?

A Final Word

The community of Parkinson's Caregivers—in person, online, and in spiritual connection—is a very special group of people. I would be very happy to hear from you, about your experience as a caregiver and, where I can, to answer questions that have come up as you've read through the chapters of *Love, Dignity, and Parkinson's*. Please feel free to reach out to me at my website, www.seaburyhouse.com. I will answer your questions if I can or help you look for resources if I don't have an answer myself.

I wish you strength, a supportive circle, and the certainty that your well-being matters as you carry on in this Parkinson's Life.

1-Click Review

Thank you for reading *Love, Dignity and Parkinson's*. Reader reviews will help to get this book into the hands of other caregivers.

If you have found the book useful to you, please take one minute to write a review on Amazon. Even a few sentences will let caregivers and other readers know about *Love, Dignity and Parkinson's*.

Scan the QR Code below to leave a review.

APPENDIX 1

Resources for Learning About Parkinson's Disease Itself

In the first chapter I suggested that you not share *Love, Dignity, and Parkinson's* with your partner, but instead to find other resources for learning about your partner's PD. Whether you and your partner have just learned about their diagnosis, or you have been walking the Parkinson's path for a long while, these resources will help you become more knowledgeable about Parkinson's.

Three Important Books

I suggest three titles that will help you and your partner to get more information about PD. If funds are tight, ask your public library to order them. Other people in your community will benefit from having them available too.

The first is *Parkinson's Disease for Dummies* (ISBN: 978-0-470-07395-7) by Michele Tagliati, Gary Guten, Jo Horne, and Deborah W. Brooks. I always suggest this excellent overview as a good place to start when a couple is looking at a new diagnosis of PD. The breezy and relaxed writing style makes this book a comfortable read, and the clear organization, little tips, and silly cartoons will let you and your PWP dip into the idea of living with PD without getting overwhelmed. You don't need to read the whole thing at once. Explore its different sections as you wish, and you will get a good overview of PD.

The second book is *The New Parkinson's Disease Treatment Book: Partnering with Your Doctor to Get the Most from Your Medications*, Second Edition by J. Eric Ahlskog, PhD, MD (2015) - Oxford: Oxford University Press. The Dummies book is the place to begin to understand the disease, but this wonderful volume, by a Mayo Clinic doctor with more than thirty years of experience in treating Parkinson's, is your guide to medical decision-making.

Read this one to learn how doctors think about medicine for Parkinson's. You'll learn more about the different treatment options, and why the plan for your partner's medicines changes over time. I used this book throughout my husband's life, and it made me much more knowledgeable about medications and treatments. It's not inexpensive (about the price of a good meal out), but in my opinion, it is worth every penny.

The third book that I found helpful is *Making the Connection Between Brain and Behavior: Coping with Parkinson's Disease* by Joseph Friedman (2013) - New York, NY: Demos Medical Pub. Increasingly, as we understand PD as a brain disease, it has become clear that the outward signs are not the first things affected by the gradual loss of dopamine that is the major feature of PD. Losing dopamine affects many other brain functions, causing changes in emotions, thinking, and behavior. Dr. Friedman's writing helped me understand more about these non-motor symptoms. Many times, it is these non-motor symptoms that make PD challenging for a caregiver. Friedman's book describes the behavioral and interpersonal changes caused by Parkinson's Disease and links them to the best available treatments.

Online Resources

There are many organizations, Facebook Groups (which are mostly private and require that you apply and be accepted), other online groups, and other web resources—far more than I can include here.

Websites

There are a number of helpful websites online to give you information about PD. Here are a few to get you started:

- Davis Phinney Foundation: https://davisphinneyfoundation.org/

- Parkinson's Disease Foundation: <u>https://www.parkinson.org/</u>

- The US National Institute on Aging offers a clear <u>overview</u> of the disease: <u>https://www.nia.nih.gov/health/parkinsons-disease#:~:text=Parkinson's%20disease%20is%20a%20brain,have%20difficulty%20walking%20and%20talking</u>.

- The Michael J. Fox Foundation: https://www.michaeljfox.org/

In Person and Online:
Support Groups and Communities

Some PWPs and their partners find time to attend in-person meetings of PD support groups in their communities. Across the country there are local support groups and organizations where PWPs and caregivers meet others with experience with PD. Your Area Office on Aging and your MDS are good places to start finding out where you and your PWP can make in-person connections for support, information, and companionship.

If the effort to attend such sessions puts this kind of help out of reach, try joining online communities. These groups vary: some require a no-cost signup and are monitored by volunteer moderators. Others are open to the general public. Most are respectful and helpful. Remember, you don't have to write anything for others to read. Sometimes just knowing that there are other caregivers out there, sharing experiences of their own, can be a real lifeline.

One such community, the Parkinson's Better Halves (pbh-org.com) website and its associated Facebook Groups, focuses specifically on the wives of men with Parkinson's and creates opportunities for community and sharing among women. Kelley Roberson, whose life partner has PD, recognized the enormous challenges of loving someone with the disease and began the PBH organization in response. I feel lucky to have joined this loving and welcoming community in learning about PD and the caregiver experience and to have been given support and encouragement in my work on this book.

Another online group, MyParkinsons.org, was started in 2001 by Jim Smitchger, a healthcare marketing company analyst and researcher, as an outgrowth of a 1999 study of Parkinson's conducted in concert with the Neurology Center at Harvard Medical School. When first launched, the MyParkinsons.org Discussion Forum was the only dedicated caregiver resource available online. This very nurturing site took on a life of its own and has maintained its important role in supporting PD Caregivers for more than twenty years. In this community, I found tremendous support during my first years in caring for my husband with Parkinson's disease. One member, in particular, Al Labendz (who wrote under the name Lohengr1n), himself had Parkinson's. His contributions to the Caregiver Discussion Forum over a seventeen-year span, until his death in 2019, were invaluable since he informed us all from his firsthand experience with the disease.

APPENDIX 2
Resources About Sexuality, Disability, and Aging

Joan Price's work is a great resource for older people to learn about sexuality. While she doesn't directly address Parkinson's in her book *Naked at our Age,* her writings are a good resource as you begin to think about how PD has affected your sexuality and your partner's. Her website has resources, blogs, and webinars that can be useful for normalizing sex as we age.

https://joanprice.com/

Other resources include:

- National Institute on Aging, which writes about the physical changes that affect sexuality as we age: *https://www.nia.nih.gov/health/sexuality-and-intimacy-older-adults#:~:text=Normal%20aging%20also%20brings%20physical,no%20longer%20find%20them%20attractive.*

- The American Psychological Association also give information on aging and human sexuality: *https://www.apa.org/pi/aging/resources/guides/sexuality*

- American Parkinson's Disease Association's page Information on Parkinson's and Sex: *https://www.apdaparkinson.org/what-is-parkinsons/symptoms/sexual-effects/?utm_content=grants&gclid=Cj0KCQjwhqaVBh-CxARIsAHKItiMTLHY_SAmcnZhoArBkjtanVs8PWnh7tOQcb0Pod-vyIe7CtY9BWd88aAic1EALw_wcB*

- Teepa Snow, who offers a wide range of information of living with and loving a partner who has dementia, also discusses sexuality and intimacy: https://teepasnow.com/blog/sexuality-and-intimacy/

APPENDIX 3
Ideas for Your Date with You

In Chapter Six I suggest that you build in a regular plan of having a date with yourself. Your date doesn't have to be elaborate. You might start by doing something simple and close to home.

For a start, visit your public library. Most have bulletin boards in the building, along with websites where they post activities and events. Maybe there is a film showing or an author may come to talk about her new book. Our public libraries are free to use, and even if you haven't been in a library since school, you'll find that the people at the desk are warm and helpful. Google "library near me" to find yours and start with their website.

As an experiment, I picked a US town at random—Emporia, Kansas (population 24,000)—and checked its public library to see what free events would be available this month:

- Book Club
- Emporia Reads together
- Mini Canvas: learn to paint a mini canvas
- Healthy cooking class: Learn to make hummus from scratch
- A presentation on pollinators and their role in our gardens
- A Craft and Chat session
- Grab and Go craft kits

Besides public libraries, many towns have local museums and historical societies. Google "museums near me" to get started.

I also checked the Emporia High School's website to see what plays and concerts were available this year. There were five shows: a musical and four plays, including an evening of one-act plays written by the school's seniors. There were also orchestra and band concerts and a drumline. You don't have to be a parent or grandparent to enjoy watching energetic youngsters spreading their artistic wings. If someone asks which child you are there to see, just give a big smile and say, "I want to see them all!"

Of course, you don't have to live in Emporia, Kansas to find free, interesting events near at hand. Do your own experiment and find out what attracts your attention. If you live near a college or university, you might look for an Osher Lifelong Living Institute in your area (https://www.osherfoundation. org/olli.html). Across the United States, the Osher Foundation supports 125 of these programs, at least one in every state. The OLLI programs are designed to focus "on the joy of learning without examinations or grades—and keeping in touch with a larger world."

A Date with You at Home

If you have to have your date at home, take advantage of the internet. Try to ignore what is familiar on YouTube or other sites, the short snippets that consume your time without giving you a satisfying experience, and skip the irritating and offensive nonsense that you might notice. It's important to avoid distraction if your date is online. Stick to your purpose: to be on a satisfying date with yourself, so that you don't get pulled into random scrolling. Stay focused and settle in for your virtual getaway!

If you want to treat yourself to a performance or concert, search *full concert* or *full performance* on YouTube to find plays, concerts, competitions that are new to you. Another good resource is the NPR Tiny Desk concerts, which are studio performances by a wide range of performers.

More formal sources for online activities include paid programs like the ones offered by Road Scholar (formerly Elderhostel) https://www.road-scholar.org/virtual-campus/ and the Open Coursewear project, which offers free college courses all around the world. https://www.merlot.org/merlot/

In addition to these suggestions, check my website (www.seaburyhouse.com) for more ideas for a date at home with yourself.